# CHRONIC KIDNEY DISEASE COOKBOOK FOR SENIORS

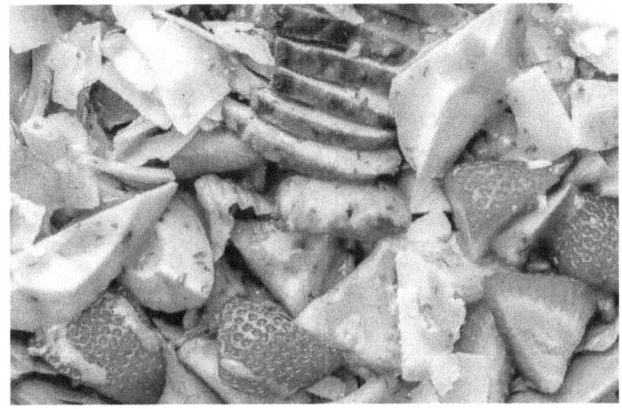

## Easy and Tasty Low Sodium, Low Potassium, and Low Phosphorus Renal Diet Recipes To Manage CKD and Avoid Dialysis, With 30 Day Meal Plan.

**Joshua S. Gray**

For more information or help feel free to contact me at:
joshuagrayhelpdesk@gmail.com

# Table of Contents

# SCAN THIS CODE TO GAIN ACCESS TO MORE BOOKS BY THE AUTHOR

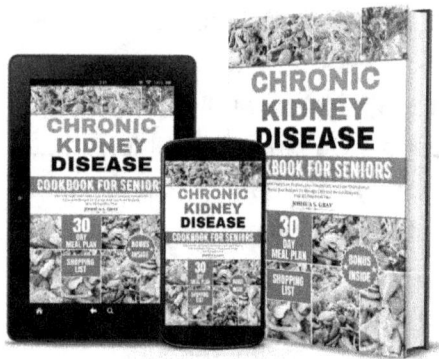

# INTRODUCTION

Have you ever considered the transformative power that lies within the meals you savor each day? Imagine embarking on a culinary adventure that will nourish your body from the inside out. Imagine for a moment a cookbook that has been painstakingly designed to revolutionize your relationship with food, particularly when navigating the nuances of health. Welcome to the "Chronic Kidney Disease Cookbook For Seniors."

Could each meal you cook be a first step toward living a more energetic, healthy life? What if cooking with purpose, rather than just using medications, was the key to managing Chronic Kidney Disease (CKD) in seniors? A journey where every recipe is a celebration of life, health, and the joy of savoring flavors awaits you as you explore the pages of this cookbook with these questions resounding through it.

Within these pages, we will take you on a special journey that combines culinary creativity with health-conscious options, designed especially for seniors living with chronic kidney disease. But this is more than just a cookbook; it's a declaration of the idea that each meal can be a nourishing step in the direction of a better, healthier future.

As we explore the core of this cookbook, you will find a variety of recipes that are not only going to please your palate but also work in perfect harmony with the dietary recommendations that are essential for seniors with chronic kidney disease. From hearty breakfasts to satisfying dinners, from delightful snacks to guilt-free desserts, each dish is a culinary masterpiece aimed at promoting kidney health without compromising on flavor.

A new outlook on health—one that finds harmony in the ingredients, balance in the flavors, and joy in the cooking process—must be adopted. This is about more than just what you eat. This cookbook transforms into your reliable companion as you pursue optimum health as it clearly explains the particular dietary requirements of seniors with CKD.

Come along with us as we explore the culinary and health domains, with each recipe serving as a new chapter in your journey toward well-being. Let's embark together on a culinary odyssey that celebrates life and nurtures health. The journey commences with the flip of a page, and as we relish the harmonious blend of tastes found in the "Chronic Kidney Disease Cookbook For Seniors."

Let the culinary journey begin. Your health deserves to be embraced with thoughtful, delicious meals.

# CHAPTER 1

## Understanding Chronic Kidney Disease (CKD)

Chronic Kidney Disease (CKD) stands as a pervasive health concern, quietly impacting millions worldwide. As we embark on an exploration of this complex condition, it becomes imperative to unravel the intricacies of its causes, symptoms, and the preventive measures that form the foundation of its management.

CKD is a progressive condition wherein the kidneys, responsible for critical functions like filtering waste and excess fluids from the blood, gradually lose their efficiency. Unlike acute kidney injury, CKD unfolds over an extended period, often remaining asymptomatic in its early stages, earning its moniker as the "silent disease."

## Causes of Chronic Kidney Disease

Numerous factors contribute to the onset and progression of CKD, with the most common being:

1.    Diabetes: Uncontrolled high blood sugar levels can lead to damage in the small blood vessels of the kidneys, impairing their ability to filter effectively.

2.    Hypertension (High Blood Pressure): Elevated blood pressure puts strain on the delicate blood vessels in the kidneys, causing gradual damage over time.

3.    Genetic    Predisposition:    Some individuals may be genetically predisposed to

kidney diseases, increasing their susceptibility to CKD.

4. **Autoimmune Disorders:** Conditions like lupus and certain infections can trigger an immune response that affects kidney function.

5. **Obesity:** Excess weight and obesity contribute to the development of diabetes and hypertension, both significant risk factors for CKD.

6. **Smoking:** Tobacco use has been linked to an increased risk of kidney damage.

7. **Age:** Aging itself is a risk factor, with kidney function naturally declining over time.

# Symptoms of Chronic Kidney Disease

CKD is often asymptomatic in its early stages, making it challenging to detect until significant kidney damage has occurred. However, as the illness worsens, a number of symptoms could show up:

1. **Fatigue:** Persistent fatigue and weakness can result from anemia, a common complication of CKD.

2. **Swelling:** Fluid retention can lead to swelling in the legs, ankles, or face.

3. **Changes in Urination:** Frequent urination, especially at night, blood in the urine, and foamy urine can be indicators of kidney dysfunction.

4. **Difficulty Concentrating:** Impaired kidney function can lead to a buildup of toxins in the blood, affecting cognitive function.

5. **Loss of Appetite:** CKD can cause a decrease in appetite and unintended weight loss.

6. **Muscle Cramps:** Electrolyte imbalances associated with CKD can result in muscle cramps.

7. **High Blood Pressure:** CKD and hypertension often create a reciprocal relationship, each exacerbating the other.

# Preventive Measures

While certain risk factors for CKD, such as age and genetics, are beyond our control, adopting proactive measures can significantly reduce the likelihood of developing this condition:

1.    **Manage Diabetes and Hypertension:** Keeping blood sugar levels and blood pressure within recommended ranges is crucial in preventing kidney damage.

2.    **Healthy Lifestyle Choices:** Maintaining a healthy weight through regular exercise and a balanced diet helps mitigate various risk factors for CKD.

3.    **Limit Salt Intake:** Excessive salt consumption can contribute to hypertension,

putting strain on the kidneys. Limiting salt intake is essential in kidney health.

4. **Stay Hydrated:** Drinking an adequate amount of water supports kidney function by helping to flush out toxins.

5. **Quit Smoking:** Smoking not only contributes to the development of CKD but also accelerates its progression. Quitting smoking is a vital step in preserving kidney health.

6. **Regular Exercise:** Engaging in regular physical activity supports overall health, helps maintain a healthy weight, and promotes cardiovascular health, reducing the risk of CKD.

7. **Moderate Alcohol Consumption:** Excessive alcohol consumption can contribute

to high blood pressure and other health issues that impact kidney function. Moderation is key.

8.    **Regular Health Check-ups:** Routine health check-ups, including monitoring blood pressure and kidney function, allow for early detection and intervention.

# CHAPTER 2

## Benefits of Following Chronic Kidney Disease Management Plan

Following a chronic kidney disease (CKD) management plan and making lifestyle changes can offer several benefits for individuals dealing with this condition. Here are some key advantages of adopting a CKD-friendly approach:

### 1. Slowing Disease Progression:

Adhering to a CKD management plan, which often includes dietary modifications, can help slow down the progression of kidney disease. Managing blood pressure, blood sugar levels, and other contributing factors can contribute to preserving kidney function.

## 2. Maintaining Optimal Nutrition:

A CKD-friendly diet emphasizes balanced nutrition while considering the restrictions necessary for kidney health. This ensures that individuals receive essential nutrients without overloading the kidneys with substances they struggle to process.

## 3. Managing Fluid Balance:

The kidneys are essential for controlling the body's fluid balance. Following a CKD management plan helps individuals manage their fluid intake, preventing excessive retention that can lead to swelling and complications.

## 4. Preventing Complications:

CKD is associated with various complications such as cardiovascular issues, anemia, and bone disorders. By managing the underlying causes and adopting a kidney-friendly lifestyle, individuals can reduce the risk of these complications.

## 5. Improved Blood Pressure Control:

High blood pressure is a common contributor to CKD progression. Lifestyle changes such as dietary modifications, regular exercise, and medication adherence can significantly contribute to better blood pressure control.

## 6. Enhancing Quality of Life:

By proactively managing CKD, individuals can experience an improved quality of life. Symptom management, reduced complications, and a sense of control over their health contribute to overall well-being.

## 7. Customized Medication Management:

Individuals with CKD often have multiple health conditions. Following a CKD management plan allows for a more customized approach to medication management, considering the potential impact on kidney function.

## 8. Preventing Malnutrition:

CKD can lead to a higher risk of malnutrition due to dietary restrictions and decreased appetite. A carefully planned CKD-friendly diet ensures that individuals receive adequate nutrition to maintain their health.

## 9. Delaying the Need for Dialysis or Transplant:

For individuals with advanced CKD, effective management may delay the need for dialysis or kidney transplant. This delay can provide individuals with more time before resorting to these more intensive interventions.

## 10. Empowering Individuals:

Following a CKD management plan empowers individuals to take an active role in their health. By understanding the impact of lifestyle choices, dietary habits, and medication adherence, individuals can feel more in control of their condition.

## 11. Supporting Mental and Emotional Well-being:

The challenges of living with a chronic condition can take a toll on mental and emotional well-being. By actively managing CKD and making positive lifestyle changes, individuals can experience a sense of accomplishment, resilience, and improved mental health.

## 12. Preventing Acute Episodes:

CKD management involves avoiding factors that can trigger acute episodes of worsening kidney function. This proactive approach helps prevent sudden declines in kidney health and the associated complications.

### 13. Education and Awareness:

Following a CKD management plan involves continuous education about the condition and its management. This increased awareness empowers individuals to make informed decisions about their health.

### 14. Collaborative Healthcare Approach:

Managing CKD often involves a collaborative approach with healthcare providers. Regular check-ups, monitoring, and adjustments to the management plan based on individual needs contribute to better health outcomes.

### 15. Encouraging Healthy Lifestyle Habits:

Adopting a CKD-friendly lifestyle often includes recommendations for regular exercise, maintaining a healthy weight, and avoiding tobacco and excessive alcohol consumption.

These habits contribute to overall health and well-being.

Following a chronic kidney disease management plan offers a holistic approach to health, addressing not only the kidney-specific concerns but also promoting overall well-being. It involves a combination of dietary adjustments, lifestyle changes, and proactive healthcare measures to enhance the quality of life for individuals living with CKD.

# Foods to Eat or Avoid

For seniors navigating the intricate landscape of Chronic Kidney Disease (CKD), dietary choices become a cornerstone in preserving and enhancing kidney health. A CKD-friendly diet is not just a culinary regimen; it's a strategic approach to nourishment that empowers seniors to achieve optimum health and well-being. Let's explore the foods to embrace and those to tread cautiously with in this delicate dietary journey.

**Foods to Eat**

**1. Low-Phosphorus Foods:**

Incorporate low-phosphorus foods to support kidney function. Examples include fresh fruits, vegetables, rice, pasta, and lean meats. These choices help manage phosphorus levels, crucial in CKD management.

## 2. Limited Sodium Intake:

Opt for fresh, whole foods and seasonings instead of relying on high-sodium processed options. Reducing sodium intake helps manage blood pressure, a pivotal aspect of CKD care.

## 3. Healthy Fats:

Select healthy fat sources such as nuts, avocados, and olive oil. These fats provide essential nutrients without contributing to the burden on the kidneys.

## 4. Moderate Protein Consumption:

Balance protein intake by choosing high-quality sources such as lean meats, fish, eggs, and dairy. Moderation is key, as excessive protein can strain the kidneys.

## 5. Fruits and Vegetables:

Embrace a rainbow of fruits and vegetables, rich in vitamins and antioxidants. These not only contribute to overall health but also offer fiber, aiding digestion and promoting heart health.

## 6. Whole Grains:

Choose whole grains such as brown rice, whole wheat bread, quinoa. These choices provide fiber, vitamins, and minerals without contributing excessive phosphorus.

## 7. Limited Potassium-Rich Foods:

While potassium is essential for health, too much can be detrimental in CKD. Choose low-potassium fruits and vegetables like apples, berries, cabbage, and green beans.

### 8. Hydration:

Prioritize hydration with water and herbal teas. Staying well-hydrated supports kidney function and helps manage fluid balance.

### 9. Calcium-Rich Foods:

Include moderate amounts of calcium-rich foods like low-fat dairy, fortified plant-based milk, and leafy greens. Adequate calcium is crucial for bone health.

### 10. Carefully Managed Dairy:

Seniors with CKD need to balance dairy intake. Choose low-fat or fat-free options and monitor phosphorus content.

**Foods to Avoid**

**1. Dairy Products:**

While dairy is a valuable source of calcium and protein, it can also be high in phosphorus. Choose lower-phosphorus options and monitor portion sizes.

**2. Nuts and Seeds:**

These are nutritious but can be high in phosphorus and potassium. Opt for smaller portions and consider them as occasional treats.

**3. Processed Foods:**

Highly processed foods often contain hidden sodium, phosphorus, and potassium. Read labels diligently and limit consumption of processed items.

## 4. Canned Foods:

Canned goods may have added sodium and phosphorus. Choose low-sodium or no-added-salt varieties, and rinse canned vegetables to reduce potassium content.

## 5. Bananas and Oranges:

While fruits are generally healthy, bananas and oranges are higher in potassium. Monitor portion sizes and consider lower-potassium alternatives.

## 6. Dried Fruits:

Dried fruits are concentrated sources of nutrients, including potassium. Consume them sparingly to manage potassium intake.

## 7. Avocado:

Avocados are rich in healthy fats but also contain potassium. Monitor portion sizes and consider them in the context of overall potassium consumption.

## 8. Red and Processed Meats:

These can be high in phosphorus and protein. Choose lean cuts, control portion sizes, and balance protein intake.

# CHAPTER 3

## Exercise as a Tool to Manage Chronic Kidney Disease For Seniors

Exercise plays a crucial role in the overall health and well-being of seniors, including those managing Chronic Kidney Disease (CKD). While individuals with CKD should approach exercise with some considerations, engaging in physical activity can bring numerous benefits. Here's a guide to exercises for seniors with CKD:

### Benefits of Exercise for Seniors with CKD:

### 1. Improved Cardiovascular Health:

Regular exercise contributes to better cardiovascular health, helping manage conditions like hypertension, a common concern in CKD.

### 2. Enhanced Muscle Strength:

Strengthening exercises help maintain and improve muscle strength, promoting overall physical function and reducing the risk of falls.

### 3. Better Weight Management:

Exercise, when combined with a healthy diet, aids in weight management. Sustaining a healthy weight is crucial for people with chronic kidney disease.

### 4. Increased Energy Levels:

Physical activity can boost energy levels and reduce fatigue, improving the overall quality of life for seniors with CKD.

### 5. Improved Mood and Mental Well-being:

Exercise has positive effects on mood and mental health. It can help alleviate stress, anxiety, and depression, common challenges faced by individuals with chronic conditions.

### 6. Enhanced Joint Flexibility:

Stretching and flexibility exercises contribute to joint health and can help seniors maintain or improve their range of motion.

### 7. Better Blood Sugar Control:

For seniors with diabetes, a common comorbidity with CKD, regular exercise can assist in better blood sugar control.

# Types of Exercise for Seniors with CKD

## 1. Aerobic Exercises:

Low-impact aerobic exercises such as walking, swimming, and cycling are generally well-tolerated by seniors with CKD. These activities improve cardiovascular health without putting excessive strain on the kidneys.

## 2. Strength Training:

Light resistance training with bands or light weights can help build and maintain muscle strength. Focus on major muscle groups but avoid heavy weights to prevent excessive strain on the kidneys.

## 3. Flexibility and Stretching Exercises:

Include activities like yoga or gentle stretching exercises to enhance flexibility. These exercises promote joint health and can be adapted to individual fitness levels.

## 4. Balance Exercises:

Balance exercises, such as standing on one leg or heel-to-toe walking, are important for preventing falls, which can be a concern for seniors.

## Considerations and Precautions:

### 1. Consultation with Healthcare Providers:

Before starting any exercise program, seniors with CKD should consult with their healthcare providers. The healthcare team can provide guidance based on the individual's health status.

### 2. Hydration:

Staying well-hydrated is crucial for individuals with CKD. Seniors should drink water before, during, and after exercise to prevent dehydration.

## 3. Monitoring Blood Pressure:

Regular monitoring of blood pressure is essential during exercise, particularly for those with hypertension. Seniors should be cautious with activities that may cause a sudden spike in blood pressure.

## 4. Avoiding Overexertion:

The advice for seniors is to listen to their bodies and refrain from doing too many of it. It's important to start slowly, gradually increasing the intensity and duration of exercise.

## 5. Adapting to Individual Abilities:

Exercises should be adapted to individual abilities and any existing health conditions. Tailoring activities to personal fitness levels ensures safety and enjoyment.

### 6. Choosing Comfortable Footwear:

Proper footwear is crucial to prevent falls and injuries. Seniors should wear comfortable, supportive shoes suitable for their chosen activities.

### 7. Incorporating Variety:

A well-rounded exercise routine includes a variety of activities to address different aspects of fitness. This can prevent boredom and provide a comprehensive approach to health.

Exercise is a valuable tool in the management of Chronic Kidney Disease for seniors. By adopting a well-rounded and individualized exercise program, seniors can enhance their physical and mental well-being, contribute to the management of CKD-related conditions, and enjoy a more active and fulfilling lifestyle. The key lies in striking a balance, consulting with healthcare professionals, and making choices that align with individual capabilities and health goals. As always, the primary goal is to empower seniors to lead healthy, active lives while managing the challenges posed by CKD.

# CHAPTER 4

## Shopping List

When shopping for a Chronic Kidney Disease (CKD) diet tailored for seniors, it's essential to focus on nutrient-dense, kidney-friendly ingredients. Here's a list of 20 items that can be included in a CKD-friendly shopping list for seniors:

### 1. Fresh Vegetables:

Opt for a variety of low-potassium vegetables such as cauliflower, bell peppers, cabbage, and green beans.

### 2. Low-Potassium Fruits:

Choose fruits like apples, berries, peaches, and plums, which are lower in potassium content.

### 3. White Bread and Pasta:

Select white bread and pasta instead of whole grain to manage phosphorus intake.

### 4. Low-Phosphorus Grains:

Include grains like white rice, couscous, and quinoa to keep phosphorus levels in check.

### 5. Lean Proteins:

Prioritize lean protein sources such as skinless poultry, fish, eggs, and tofu. These provide essential nutrients without excessive phosphorus.

### 6. Low-Fat Dairy:

Opt for low-fat or fat-free dairy products like milk, yogurt, and cheese to manage phosphorus and saturated fat intake.

### 7. Herbs and Spices:

Use herbs and spices like garlic, onion, basil, and oregano to flavor meals without adding sodium.

### 8. Olive Oil:

Choose olive oil as a healthy fat alternative to contribute to heart health.

### 9. Low-Sodium Canned Goods:

When using canned goods, select low-sodium or no-added-salt varieties, such as low-sodium canned vegetables or beans.

### 10. Fresh Herbs:

Include fresh herbs like parsley, cilantro, and dill to add flavor without additional sodium.

## 11. Low-Potassium Snack Options:

Consider snacks like popcorn, rice cakes, and pretzels as lower-potassium alternatives.

## 12. Low-Phosphorus Nuts:

Include nuts with lower phosphorus content, such as almonds and cashews, in moderation.

## 13. Low-Potassium Cooking Ingredients:

Use low-potassium cooking ingredients like vinegar, lemon juice, and mustard for added flavor.

## 14. Ground Turkey or Chicken:

Lean ground turkey or chicken is a protein-rich option with lower phosphorus content.

## 15. Fresh Eggs:

Eggs are a versatile and kidney-friendly protein source.

### 16. Low-Potassium Berries:

Berries like strawberries, blueberries, and raspberries are not only delicious but also lower in potassium.

### 17. Unsalted Butter:

Choose unsalted butter or consider using healthy alternatives like olive oil in cooking.

### 18. Low-Phosphorus Breakfast Cereals:

Look for low-phosphorus breakfast cereals fortified with essential vitamins and minerals.

### 19. Low-Potassium Beverages:

Include beverages like herbal teas, coffee, and cranberry juice (in moderation) to stay hydrated without excess potassium.

### 20. Low-Phosphorus Dessert Options:

Consider desserts with lower phosphorus content, such as sorbet, angel food cake, or homemade cookies using kidney-friendly ingredients.

# Shopping Tips

### 1. Read Labels:

Pay attention to food labels, especially regarding potassium and phosphorus content.

### 2. Fresh vs. Processed:

Prioritize fresh, whole foods over processed options to reduce sodium, phosphorus, and potassium intake.

### 3. Portion Control:

Practice portion control to manage nutrient intake effectively.

### 4. Plan Meals:

Plan meals in advance to ensure a balanced and kidney-friendly diet.

## 5. Stay Hydrated:

Include hydrating options like water, herbal teas, and diluted fruit juices.

## 6. Variety is Key:

Ensure a variety of foods to obtain a range of essential nutrients.

By focusing on these kidney-friendly ingredients and incorporating them into well-balanced meals, seniors with CKD can enjoy a flavorful and nourishing diet that supports their overall health and well-being.

# CHAPTER 5

# Breakfast Recipes

## 1. Apple Cinnamon Overnight Oats

Ingredients:

- ½ cup rolled oats

- ½ cup low-fat milk or a dairy-free alternative

- ½ medium apple, diced

- ½ teaspoon cinnamon

- 1 tablespoon of chopped nuts like walnuts or almonds

Preparation:

1. In a jar or container, combine rolled oats, milk, diced apple, and cinnamon.

2. Stir well, cover, and refrigerate overnight.

3. Before serving, top with chopped nuts.

**Nutritional Value:**

- Calories: Approximately 300

- Protein: 10g

- Fiber: 6g

- Potassium: 200mg

## 2.   Egg Drop Soup

**Ingredients:**

- 2 cups of vegetable broth or low-sodium chicken
- 1 large egg, beaten
- 1 green onion, thinly sliced
- ¼ teaspoon ginger, grated
- ¼ teaspoon low-sodium soy sauce

**Preparation:**

1. Bring the broth to a simmer in a pot.

2. Slowly pour in the beaten egg while stirring the soup.

3. Add sliced green onions, grated ginger, and soy sauce.

4. Cook for an additional 2-3 minutes.

**Nutritional Value:**

- Calories: Approximately 80

- Protein: 7g

- Sodium: 150mg

## 3. Ham and Cheese Omelet

Ingredients:

- 2 large eggs

- 2 slices low-sodium ham, diced

- ¼ cup low-fat shredded cheese

- Salt and pepper to taste

- 1 teaspoon olive oil


Preparation:

1. Beat eggs in a bowl and season with salt and pepper.

2. A skillet with medium heat should be used to heat the olive oil.

3. Pour the beaten eggs into the pan, add diced ham and cheese.

4. Cook until the edges are set, then fold the omelet in half.

**Nutritional Value:**

- Calories: Approximately 250

- Protein: 20g

- Sodium: 300mg

# 4.   Greek Yogurt with Honey and Nuts

Ingredients:

- ½ cup plain Greek yogurt

- 1 tablespoon honey

- 1 tablespoon of chopped nuts like walnuts or almonds

Preparation:

1. Spoon Greek yogurt into a bowl.

2. Drizzle honey over the yogurt.

3. Sprinkle chopped nuts on top.

Nutritional Value:

- Calories: Approximately 200

- Protein: 15g

- Potassium: 150mg

## 5.   Berry Smoothie

**Ingredients:**

- ½ cup mixed strawberries, blueberries, and raspberries
- ½ banana
- ½ cup low-fat milk or a dairy-free alternative
- ½ cup ice cubes

**Preparation:**

1. Blend all ingredients until smooth.
2. Adjust thickness with more liquid if needed.

**Nutritional Value:**

- Calories: Approximately 150
- Protein: 5g
- Fiber: 4g

# 6. Veggie Breakfast Burrito

Ingredients:

- 1 whole wheat tortilla
- 2 eggs, scrambled
- ¼ cup black beans, drained and rinsed
- ¼ cup diced tomatoes
- 2 tablespoons diced bell peppers
- 1 tablespoon chopped cilantro
- Salsa (optional)

Preparation:

1. Fill the tortilla with scrambled eggs, black beans, tomatoes, bell peppers, and cilantro.
2. Roll into a burrito and, if desired, serve with salsa.

Nutritional Value:

- Calories: Approximately 300
- Protein: 15g
- Fiber: 6g

## 7.  Easy Turnip Puree

**Ingredients:**

- 2 medium turnips, peeled and diced

- 1 tablespoon olive oil

- Salt and pepper to taste

- 1 tablespoon chopped chives (optional)

**Preparation:**

1. Boil or steam diced turnips until fork-tender.

2. Mash the turnips, adding olive oil, salt, and pepper.

3. Garnish with chopped chives if desired.

**Nutritional Value:**

- Calories: Approximately 100

- Fiber: 4g

- Potassium: 200mg

# 8.   Cinnamon Apple Cakes

**Ingredients:**

- ½ cup oat flour
- ½ teaspoon baking powder
- ¼ teaspoon cinnamon
- ½ medium apple, grated
- 1 egg
- ¼ cup low-fat milk or a dairy-free alternative
- 1 tablespoon honey

**Preparation:**

1. In a bowl, mix oat flour, baking powder, and cinnamon.

2. Add grated apple, egg, milk, and honey. Mix until well combined.

3. After greasing a muffin tin, pour the batter inside.

4. Bake in a preheated oven at 350°F (180°C) for about 15-20 minutes.

**Nutritional Value:**

- Calories: Approximately 150
- Protein: 5g
- Fiber: 3g

# 9. Oatmeal with Fresh Berries

**Ingredients:**

- ½ cup rolled oats
- 1 cup water or low-fat milk
- ½ cup mixed strawberries, blueberries, and raspberries
- 1 tablespoon of chopped nuts like walnuts and almonds

**Preparation:**

1. Cook rolled oats in water or milk according to package instructions.
2. Top with mixed berries and chopped nuts before serving.

**Nutritional Value:**

- Calories: Approximately 200
- Protein: 6g
- Fiber: 5g

# 10. Egg and Vegetable Muffins

**Ingredients:**

- 4 eggs
- ¼ cup diced bell peppers
- ¼ cup diced tomatoes
- 2 tablespoons chopped spinach
- Salt and pepper to taste

**Preparation:**

1. Preheat the oven to 350°F (180°C).
2. Whisk eggs in a bowl and add diced vegetables, salt, and pepper.
3. Pour the mixture into greased muffin cups.
4. Bake for 15-20 minutes until set.

**Nutritional Value:**

- Calories: Approximately 150
- Protein: 10g

# CHAPTER 6

# Lunch Recipes

## 1. Roasted Salmon with Dill

Ingredients:

- 1 salmon fillet (about 4-6 ounces)

- 1 tablespoon olive oil

- Fresh dill (to taste)

- Lemon slices for garnish

- Salt and pepper to taste

Preparation:

1. Preheat the oven to 400°F (200°C).

2. Place salmon on a baking sheet, drizzle with olive oil, and season with pepper, salt, and fresh dill.

3. Roast for about 15-20 minutes until the salmon is cooked through.

4. Garnish with lemon slices before serving.

**Nutritional Value:**

- Calories: Approximately 250

- Protein: 25g

- Omega-3 Fatty Acids: High

## 2.  Broccoli Chicken Stir Fry

Ingredients:

- 1 cup broccoli florets

- 4 ounces chicken breast, sliced

- 1 tablespoon low-sodium soy sauce

- 1 tablespoon olive oil

- 1 clove garlic, minced

- Ginger (to taste)

- Sesame seeds for garnish

Preparation:

1. A skillet with medium heat should be used to heat the olive oil.

2. Add sliced chicken and cook until browned.

3. Add broccoli, minced garlic, and ginger. Stir-fry until broccoli is tender.

4. Drizzle with soy sauce and cook for an additional 2-3 minutes.

5. Garnish with sesame seeds before serving.

**Nutritional Value:**

- Calories: Approximately 300

- Protein: 25g

- Fiber: 3g

# 3. Greek Style Roasted Vegetables

**Ingredients:**

- 2 cups mixed vegetables (zucchini, bell peppers, cherry tomatoes)
- 1 tablespoon olive oil
- 1 teaspoon dried oregano
- Feta cheese for garnish (optional)
- Salt and pepper to taste

**Preparation:**

1. Preheat the oven to 400°F (200°C).
2. Toss mixed vegetables with olive oil, dried oregano, salt, and pepper.
3. Roast for about 20-25 minutes until vegetables are tender.
4. Garnish with feta cheese before serving.

**Nutritional Value:**

- Calories: Approximately 150
- Fiber: 5g

## 4.   Beef Brisket

**Ingredients:**

- 4 ounces beef brisket

- 1 tablespoon olive oil

- ½ cup low-sodium beef broth

- 1 teaspoon garlic powder

- 1 teaspoon onion powder

- Salt and pepper to taste

**Preparation:**

1. Preheat the oven to 325°F (160°C).

2. Rub beef brisket with garlic powder, onion powder, salt, and pepper.

3. Heat olive oil in an oven-safe pan, sear brisket on all sides.

4. Add beef broth, cover, and bake for about 2-3 hours until tender.

**Nutritional Value:**

- Calories: Approximately 300

- Protein: 30g

# 5. Vegetarian Gobi Curry

**Ingredients:**

- 2 cups cauliflower florets
- 1 cup peas
- 1 cup diced tomatoes
- 1 onion, finely chopped
- 1 tablespoon olive oil
- 1 teaspoon curry powder
- Cilantro for garnish
- Salt and pepper to taste

**Preparation:**

1. Heat olive oil in a pan, sauté chopped onion until golden.

2. Add diced tomatoes, cauliflower, peas, curry powder, salt, and pepper.

3. Cook until vegetables are tender.

4. Garnish with cilantro before serving.

**Nutritional Value:**

- Calories: Approximately 200

- Protein: 7g

- Fiber: 8g

# 6. Grilled Vegetable Skewers

**Ingredients:**

- 1 zucchini, sliced

- 1 bell pepper, diced

- 1 red onion, sliced

- Cherry tomatoes

- 1 tablespoon olive oil

- 1 teaspoon Italian seasoning

- Balsamic glaze for drizzling

- Salt and pepper to taste

**Preparation:**

1. Preheat the grill.

2. Thread vegetables onto skewers, brush with olive oil, and sprinkle with Italian seasoning, salt, and pepper.

3. Grill for about 10-15 minutes until vegetables are cooked.

4. Drizzle with balsamic glaze before serving.

**Nutritional Value:**

- Calories: Approximately 150

- Fiber: 5g

# 7.   Lentil and Vegetable Curry

Ingredients:

- ½ cup lentils (rinsed and drained)

- 1 cup mixed vegetables (carrots, bell peppers, peas)

- 1 onion, finely chopped

- 1 clove garlic, minced

- 1 tablespoon olive oil

- 1 teaspoon curry powder

- Coconut milk (optional)

- Salt and pepper to taste


Preparation:

1.  Cook lentils according to package instructions.

2. In a separate pan, sauté chopped onion and garlic in olive oil until softened.

3. Add mixed vegetables, curry powder, cooked lentils, and coconut milk if desired.

4. Cook until vegetables are tender.

Nutritional Value:

- Calories: Approximately 250
- Protein: 15g
- Fiber: 10g

# 8.   Grilled Lemon Herb Tofu

Ingredients:

- 6 ounces firm tofu, sliced

- 1 tablespoon olive oil

- 1 tablespoon lemon juice

- Fresh herbs (such as thyme or rosemary)

- Salt and pepper to taste

Preparation:

1. Mix olive oil, lemon juice, fresh herbs, salt, and pepper in a bowl.

2. Marinate tofu slices in the mixture for at least 30 minutes.

3. Grill tofu for about 3-4 minutes on each side.

Nutritional Value:

- Calories: Approximately 200

- Protein: 15g

# 9. Baked Cod with Lemon and Herb

Ingredients:

- 1 cod fillet (about 4-6 ounces)

- 1 tablespoon olive oil

- 1 tablespoon lemon juice

- Fresh herbs (such as parsley or dill)

- Salt and pepper to taste

Preparation:

1. Preheat the oven to 400°F (200°C).

2. Place cod fillet on a baking sheet, drizzle with olive oil, lemon juice, and season with salt, pepper, and fresh herbs.

3. Bake for about 15-20 minutes until the cod is cooked through.

Nutritional Value:

- Calories: Approximately 200

- Protein: 25g

# 10.  Grilled Turkey Burgers

**Ingredients:**

- 4 ounces ground turkey
- 1 teaspoon olive oil
- ½ teaspoon garlic powder
- ½ teaspoon onion powder
- Whole wheat burger bun
- Lettuce, tomato, and onion slices for topping

**Preparation:**

1. In a bowl, mix ground turkey with olive oil, garlic powder, and onion powder.

2. Form the mixture into a patty.

3. Grill the turkey patty for about 5-7 minutes on each side.

4. Serve on a whole wheat bun with lettuce, tomato, and onion.

**Nutritional Value:**

- Calories: Approximately 250

- Protein: 20g

# CHAPTER 7

# Dinner Recipes

## 1. Turkey and Vegetable Skillet

Ingredients:

- 4 ounces ground turkey

- 1 tablespoon olive oil

- 1 cup mixed vegetables (bell peppers, zucchini, carrots)

- 1 teaspoon Italian seasoning

- Salt and pepper to taste

Preparation:

1. In a skillet, brown ground turkey in olive oil.

2. Add mixed vegetables and cook until tender.

3. Season with Italian seasoning, pepper, and salt.

**Nutritional Value:**

- Calories: Approximately 300

- Protein: 20g

- Fiber: 5g

## 2.   Beef Kabobs with Pepper

Ingredients:

- 4 ounces lean beef, cut into cubes

- Bell peppers, cut into chunks

- 1 tablespoon olive oil

- 1 teaspoon garlic powder

- 1 teaspoon paprika

- Salt and pepper to taste

Preparation:

1. Preheat the grill.

2. Thread beef and bell peppers onto skewers.

3. Brush with olive oil and season with garlic powder, paprika, salt, and pepper.

4. Grill for about 10-15 minutes, turning occasionally.

Nutritional Value:

- Calories: Approximately 250

- Protein: 25g

## 3. Baked Cod with Lemon Caper Sauce

Ingredients:

- 1 cod fillet (about 4-6 ounces)
- 1 tablespoon olive oil
- 1 tablespoon lemon juice
- 1 tablespoon capers
- Fresh parsley for garnish
- Salt and pepper to taste

Preparation:

1. Preheat the oven to 400°F (200°C).

2. Place cod fillet on a baking sheet, drizzle with olive oil, lemon juice, and season with salt and pepper.

3. Bake for about 15-20 minutes until the cod is cooked through.

4. Top with capers and fresh parsley before serving.

**Nutritional Value:**

- Calories: Approximately 200
- Protein: 25g

## 4. Lemon Garlic Shrimp Skewers

### Ingredients:

- 6 large shrimp, peeled and deveined
- 1 tablespoon olive oil
- 1 clove garlic, minced
- 1 tablespoon lemon juice
- Fresh parsley for garnish
- Salt and pepper to taste

### Preparation:

1. Preheat the grill.
2. Thread shrimp onto skewers.
3. Mix olive oil, minced garlic, lemon juice, salt, and pepper.
4. Brush the mixture over shrimp.
5. Grill for about 2-3 minutes on each side.
6. Garnish with fresh parsley before serving.

**Nutritional Value:**

- Calories: Approximately 150

- Protein: 20g

# 5. Grilled Balsamic Pork Chops

## Ingredients:

- 2 boneless pork chops
- 1 tablespoon balsamic vinegar
- 1 tablespoon olive oil
- 1 teaspoon dried thyme
- Salt and pepper to taste

## Preparation:

1. Preheat the grill.

2. Mix balsamic vinegar, olive oil, dried thyme, salt, and pepper.

3. Marinate pork chops in the mixture for at least 30 minutes.

4. Grill for about 5-7 minutes on each side.

## Nutritional Value:

- Calories: Approximately 300
- Protein: 30g

# 6. Spinach and Mushroom Omelet

## Ingredients:

- 2 eggs

- 1 cup fresh spinach

- ½ cup sliced mushrooms

- 1 tablespoon olive oil

- 1 tablespoon feta cheese

- Salt and pepper to taste

## Preparation:

1. In a pan, sauté spinach and mushrooms in olive oil until wilted.

2. Whisk eggs and pour over the vegetables.

3. Cook until the eggs are set.

4. Sprinkle with feta cheese before serving.

## Nutritional Value:

- Calories: Approximately 250

- Protein: 15g

# 7. Vegetable Stir Fry with Shrimp

Ingredients:

- 6 large shrimp, peeled and deveined

- 1 cup mixed vegetables (broccoli, snap peas, bell peppers)

- 1 tablespoon low-sodium soy sauce

- 1 tablespoon olive oil

- 1 teaspoon ginger, grated

- Sesame seeds for garnish

Preparation:

1. A skillet with medium heat should be used to heat the olive oil.

2. Add shrimp and cook until pink.

3. Add mixed vegetables and grated ginger, stir-fry until vegetables are tender.

4. Drizzle with soy sauce and cook for an additional 2-3 minutes.

5. Garnish with sesame seeds before serving.

**Nutritional Value:**

- Calories: Approximately 200
- Protein: 20g
- Fiber: 5g

## 8.  Beer Pork Ribs

**Ingredients:**

- 4 ounces pork ribs

- ½ cup beer (choose a low-alcohol option)

- 1 tablespoon olive oil

- 1 teaspoon smoked paprika

- Salt and pepper to taste

**Preparation:**

1. Preheat the oven to 325°F (160°C).

2. Rub pork ribs with smoked paprika, salt, and pepper.

3. Place ribs in a baking dish, pour beer over the top, and drizzle with olive oil.

4. Cover with foil and bake for about 2-3 hours until tender.

**Nutritional Value:**

- Calories: Approximately 300

- Protein: 20g

# 9. Baked Cod with Roasted Vegetables

Ingredients:

- 1 cod fillet (about 4-6 ounces)
- 1 tablespoon olive oil
- 1 cup mixed vegetables (zucchini, cherry tomatoes, bell peppers)
- 1 teaspoon dried thyme
- Salt and pepper to taste

Preparation:

1. Preheat the oven to 400°F (200°C).
2. Place cod fillet on a baking sheet, drizzle with olive oil, and season with dried thyme, salt, and pepper.
3. Surround the cod with mixed vegetables.
4. Bake for about 15-20 minutes until the cod is cooked through.

**Nutritional Value:**

- Calories: Approximately 200

- Protein: 25g

- Fiber: 5g

# 10. Shrimp and Asparagus Stir Fry

Ingredients:

- 6 large shrimp, peeled and deveined
- 1 cup asparagus spears, chopped
- 1 tablespoon low-sodium soy sauce
- 1 tablespoon olive oil
- 1 teaspoon garlic, minced
- Sesame seeds for garnish

Preparation:

1. A skillet with medium heat should be used to heat the olive oil.

2. Add shrimp and cook until pink.

3. Add asparagus and minced garlic, stir-fry until asparagus is tender.

4. Drizzle with soy sauce and cook for an additional 2-3 minutes.

5. Garnish with sesame seeds before serving.

**Nutritional Value:**

- Calories: Approximately 150
- Protein: 20g

# CHAPTER 8

## Snack Recipes

### 1.   Carrot and Ginger Soup

Ingredients:

- 2 cups carrots, chopped

- 1 tablespoon olive oil

- 1 teaspoon ginger, grated

- 4 cups low-sodium vegetable broth

- Salt and pepper to taste

Preparation:

1. In a pot, sauté chopped carrots and grated ginger in olive oil.

2. Add vegetable broth, bring to a boil, then simmer until carrots are tender.

3. Blend until smooth using a blender or immersion blender.

4. Season with pepper and salt before serving.

**Nutritional Value:**

- Calories: Approximately 100

- Fiber: 4g

## 2.   Cucumber Roll-Ups

- 1 cucumber, thinly sliced lengthwise

- 4 ounces low-sodium deli turkey or chicken slices

- ¼ cup hummus

- Fresh herbs (such as parsley or dill)


Preparation:

1. Lay cucumber slices flat and spread hummus on each slice.

2. Place turkey or chicken slices on top.

3. Roll up the cucumber slices.

4. Secure with toothpicks and garnish with fresh herbs.


Nutritional Value:

- Calories: Approximately 150

- Protein: 10g

## 3.    Baked Eggplant Chips

**Ingredients:**

- 1 medium eggplant, thinly sliced

- 2 tablespoons olive oil

- 1 teaspoon Italian seasoning

- Salt and pepper to taste

**Preparation:**

1. Preheat the oven to 375°F (190°C).

2. Toss eggplant slices in olive oil, Italian seasoning, salt, and pepper.

3. Arrange slices on a baking sheet and bake for about 15-20 minutes until crispy.

**Nutritional Value:**

- Calories: Approximately 100

- Fiber: 5g

# 4. Blueberry Oat Muffins

Ingredients:

- 1 cup oats
- ½ cup blueberries
- 2 ripe bananas, mashed
- 2 eggs
- 1 teaspoon baking powder
- 1 teaspoon vanilla extract

Preparation:

1. Preheat the oven to 350°F (180°C).

2. In a bowl, mix oats, blueberries, mashed bananas, eggs, baking powder, and vanilla extract.

3. Pour the batter into a muffin tin and bake for about 20-25 minutes.

**Nutritional Value:**

- Calories: Approximately 150
- Protein: 5g
- Fiber: 4g

# 5.   Zucchini and Corn Fritters

Ingredients:

- 1 cup grated zucchini
- ½ cup corn kernels
- ¼ cup whole wheat flour
- 1 egg
- 1 tablespoon olive oil
- ½ teaspoon garlic powder
- Salt and pepper to taste

Preparation:

1. In a bowl, combine grated zucchini, corn kernels, whole wheat flour, egg, garlic powder, salt, and pepper.

2. A skillet with medium heat should be used to heat the olive oil.

3. Spoon the mixture into the pan to form fritters and cook on each side until golden brown.

Nutritional Value:

- Calories: Approximately 150
- Protein: 6g
- Fiber: 3g

# 6.   Turkey Lettuce Wraps

Ingredients:

- 4 large lettuce leaves

- 4 ounces low-sodium deli turkey slices

- ½ cup cherry tomatoes, halved

- ¼ cup cucumber, diced

- Mustard or low-sodium dressing for drizzling

Preparation:

1. Lay out lettuce leaves.

2. Place turkey slices on each leaf.

3. Add cherry tomatoes and diced cucumber.

4. Drizzle with mustard or low-sodium dressing before rolling up.

Nutritional Value:

- Calories: Approximately 200

- Protein: 15g

# 7. Baked Sweet Potato Chips

- 1 sweet potato, thinly sliced
- 2 tablespoons olive oil
- ½ teaspoon paprika
- Salt to taste

Preparation:

1. Preheat the oven to 375°F (190°C).

2. Toss sweet potato slices in olive oil, paprika, and salt.

3. Arrange slices on a baking sheet and bake for about 15-20 minutes until crispy.

Nutritional Value:

- Calories: Approximately 150
- Fiber: 4g

# 8.   Egg Salad Lettuce Wraps

**Ingredients:**

- 2 hard-boiled eggs, chopped

- 1 tablespoon Greek yogurt

- 1 teaspoon Dijon mustard

- 4 large lettuce leaves

- Salt and pepper to taste

**Preparation:**

1. In a bowl, mix chopped hard-boiled eggs, Greek yogurt, Dijon mustard, salt, and pepper.

2. Spoon the egg salad onto lettuce leaves.

3. Roll up the lettuce leaves to form wraps.

**Nutritional Value:**

- Calories: Approximately 200

- Protein: 12g

# 9. Cucumber and Yoghurt Dip

## Ingredients:

- 1 cucumber, diced
- 1 cup Greek yogurt
- 1 tablespoon fresh dill, chopped
- 1 clove garlic, minced
- Salt and pepper to taste

## Preparation:

1. In a bowl, mix diced cucumber, Greek yogurt, chopped dill, minced garlic, salt, and pepper.
2. Chill in the refrigerator before serving.

## Nutritional Value:

- Calories: Approximately 100
- Protein: 10g

# 10. Apple and Almond Butter Wraps

### Ingredients:

- 1 apple, thinly sliced
- 2 tablespoons almond butter
- 4 whole wheat tortillas
- Cinnamon for sprinkling (optional)

### Preparation:

1. Spread almond butter on each whole wheat tortilla.
2. Place apple slices on top.
3. Sprinkle with cinnamon if desired.
4. Roll up the tortillas to form wraps.

### Nutritional Value:

- Calories: Approximately 250
- Protein: 6g
- Fiber: 5g

# CHAPTER 9

# Dessert Recipes

## 1.  Lemon Yoghurt Cake

Ingredients:

- 1 cup whole wheat flour

- ½ cup Greek yoghurt

- ¼ cup olive oil

- ½ cup honey

- 2 eggs

- 1 teaspoon baking powder

- Zest of 1 lemon

- Juice of 1 lemon

**Preparation:**

1. Preheat the oven to 350°F (180°C).

2. In a bowl, whisk together flour, Greek yoghurt, olive oil, honey, eggs, baking powder, lemon zest, and lemon juice.

3. Pour the batter into a greased baking pan.

4. Bake for about 25-30 minutes until a toothpick inserted comes out clean.

**Nutritional Value:**

- Calories: Approximately 200
- Protein: 5g

## 2.   Cinnamon Rice Cakes

**Ingredients:**

- 2 rice cakes

- 1 tablespoon almond butter

- ½ teaspoon ground cinnamon

- 1 teaspoon honey (optional)

**Preparation:**

1. Spread almond butter on rice cakes.

2. Sprinkle ground cinnamon on top.

3. Drizzle with honey if desired.

**Nutritional Value:**

- Calories: Approximately 150

- Protein: 3g

# 3.   Chocolate Mousse

Ingredients:

- 1 ripe avocado
- ¼ cup cocoa powder
- ¼ cup honey
- 1 teaspoon vanilla extract
- ¼ cup almond milk

Preparation:

1. Blend avocado, cocoa powder, honey, vanilla extract, and almond milk until smooth.
2. Chill in the refrigerator before serving.

Nutritional Value:

- Calories: Approximately 200
- Protein: 3g

# 4. Pears with Honey and Cinnamon

## Ingredients:

- 2 pears, sliced
- 1 tablespoon honey
- ½ teaspoon ground cinnamon

## Preparation:

1. Arrange pear slices on a plate.
2. Drizzle with honey and sprinkle with ground cinnamon.

## Nutritional Value:

- Calories: Approximately 100
- Fiber: 6g

# 5. Pineapple Coconut Smoothie

### Ingredients:

- 1 cup pineapple chunks
- ½ cup coconut milk
- ½ cup Greek yoghurt
- Ice cubes (optional)

### Preparation:

1. Blend pineapple chunks, coconut milk, Greek yoghurt, and ice cubes until smooth.

### Nutritional Value:

- Calories: Approximately 150
- Protein: 4g

# 6.    Raspberry Chia Jam

Ingredients:

- 1 cup raspberries
- 2 tablespoons chia seeds
- 1 tablespoon honey

Preparation:

1. Mash raspberries in a bowl.

2. Stir in chia seeds and honey.

3. Let it sit in the refrigerator until it thickens.

Nutritional Value:

- Calories: Approximately 80
- Fiber: 8g

# 7.   Carrot Cake Muffins

**Ingredients:**

- 1 cup grated carrots
- ½ cup almond flour
- ¼ cup coconut flour
- ¼ cup honey
- 2 eggs
- ½ teaspoon baking soda
- ½ teaspoon ground cinnamon

**Preparation:**

1. Preheat the oven to 350°F (180°C).

2. In a bowl, mix grated carrots, almond flour, coconut flour, honey, eggs, baking soda, and ground cinnamon.

3. Pour the batter into muffin cups.

4. Bake for about 20-25 minutes until a toothpick inserted comes out clean.

**Nutritional Value:**

- Calories: Approximately 150
- Protein: 5g

# 8.   Peach Crumble

- 2 peaches, sliced
- ¼ cup oats
- 2 tablespoons almond flour
- 1 tablespoon honey
- ½ teaspoon ground cinnamon

Preparation:

1. Preheat the oven to 375°F (190°C).

2. In a bowl, toss peach slices with oats, almond flour, honey, and ground cinnamon.

3. Transfer to a baking dish and bake for about 20-25 minutes until the top is golden.

Nutritional Value:

- Calories: Approximately 150
- Fiber: 4g

# 9. Honeydew Lime Sorbet

**Ingredients:**

- 2 cups honeydew melon, cubed
- Juice of 2 limes
- 2 tablespoons honey
- Mint leaves for garnish

**Preparation:**

1. Blend honeydew melon, lime juice, and honey until smooth.
2. Pour into a shallow dish and freeze.
3. Scoop into bowls and garnish with mint leaves before serving.

**Nutritional Value:**

- Calories: Approximately 100
- Fiber: 2g

# 10. Strawberry Frozen Yoghurt

**Ingredients:**

- 1 cup frozen strawberries
- ½ cup Greek yoghurt
- 1 tablespoon honey
- ½ teaspoon vanilla extract

**Preparation:**

1. Blend frozen strawberries, Greek yoghurt, honey, and vanilla extract until smooth.
2. Freeze for a few hours before serving.

**Nutritional Value:**

- Calories: Approximately 150
- Protein: 5g

# 30 Day Meal Plan

## Week 1

### Day 1:

Breakfast: Berry Smoothie

Lunch: Grilled Lemon Herb Tofu with Roasted Vegetables

Dinner: Lemon Garlic Shrimp Skewers with Quinoa Salad

Snack: Cucumber Roll-Ups

Dessert: Cinnamon Rice Cakes

### Day 2:

Breakfast: Greek Yogurt with Honey and Nuts

Lunch: Chickpea Salad with Vegetables

Dinner: Baked Cod with Lemon Caper Sauce and Herb Cauliflower Rice

Snack: Blueberry Oat Muffins

Dessert: Pineapple Coconut Smoothie

Day 3:

Breakfast: Oatmeal with Fresh Berries

Lunch: Shrimp Noodles with Veggies

Dinner: Spinach and Mushroom Omelet

Snack: Baked Sweet Potato Chips

Dessert: Chocolate Mousse

Day 4:

Breakfast: Veggie Breakfast Burrito

Lunch: Fusilli Salad with Avocado

Dinner: Turkey and Vegetable Skillet

Snack: Zucchini and Corn Fritters

Dessert: Pears with Honey and Cinnamon

Day 5:

Breakfast: Cinnamon Apple Cakes

Lunch: Tuna Salad with Feta Cheese and Spinach

Dinner: Grilled Balsamic Pork Chops with Greek Style Stuffed Mushrooms

Snack: Raspberry Chia Jam

Dessert: Carrot Cake Muffins

## Day 6:

Breakfast: Egg and Vegetable Muffins

Lunch: Fresh Pasta Salad with Vegetables

Dinner: Lemon Yoghurt Cake

Snack: Turkey Lettuce Wraps

Dessert: Peach Crumble

## Day 7:

Breakfast: Apple Cinnamon Overnight Oat

Lunch: Delicious Cod Sandwich

Dinner: Shrimp and Asparagus Stir Fry with Herb Cauliflower Rice

Snack: Chocolate Banana Morsels

Dessert: Honeydew Lime Sorbet

# Week 2

Breakfast: Toast with Avocado and Eggs

Lunch: Grilled Vegetable Skewers

Dinner: Pasta with Beef

Snack: Blueberry and Oat Cake

Dessert: Strawberry Frozen Yoghurt

Breakfast: Baked Eggs with Veggies

Lunch: Easy Quinoa Salad

Dinner: Beef Kabobs with Pepper

Snack: Apple and Almond Butter Wraps

Dessert: Lemon Yoghurt Cake

Day 10:

Breakfast: Ham and Cheese Omelet

Lunch: Seafood Pasta with Tomatoes

Dinner: Baked Cod with Roasted Vegetables

Snack: Carrot and Ginger Soup

Dessert: Strawberry Frozen Yoghurt


Day 11:

Breakfast: Egg and Vegetable Muffins

Lunch: Fresh Pasta Salad with Vegetables

Dinner: Lemon Yoghurt Cake

Snack: Turkey Lettuce Wraps

Dessert: Peach Crumble


Day 12:

Breakfast: Apple Cinnamon Overnight Oat

Lunch: Delicious Cod Sandwich

Dinner: Shrimp and Asparagus Stir Fry with Herb Cauliflower Rice

Snack: Chocolate Banana Morsels

Dessert: Honeydew Lime Sorbet

Day 13:

Breakfast: Toast with Avocado and Eggs

Lunch: Grilled Vegetable Skewers

Dinner: Pasta with Beef

Snack: Blueberry and Oat Cake

Dessert: Strawberry Frozen Yoghurt

Day 14:

Breakfast: Baked Eggs with Veggies

Lunch: Easy Quinoa Salad

Dinner: Beef Kabobs with Pepper

Snack: Apple and Almond Butter Wraps

Dessert: Lemon Yoghurt Cake

# Week 3

Breakfast: Ham and Cheese Omelet

Lunch: Seafood Pasta with Tomatoes

Dinner: Baked Cod with Roasted Vegetables

Snack: Carrot and Ginger Soup

Dessert: Strawberry Frozen Yoghurt

Breakfast: Berry Smoothie

Lunch: Grilled Lemon Herb Tofu with Roasted Vegetables

Dinner: Lemon Garlic Shrimp Skewers with Quinoa Salad

Snack: Cucumber Roll-Ups

Dessert: Cinnamon Rice Cakes

Day 17:

Breakfast: Greek Yogurt with Honey and Nuts

Lunch: Chickpea Salad with Vegetables

Dinner: Baked Cod with Lemon Caper Sauce and Herb Cauliflower Rice

Snack: Blueberry Oat Muffins

Dessert: Pineapple Coconut Smoothie

Day 18:

Breakfast: Oatmeal with Fresh Berries

Lunch: Shrimp Noodles with Veggies

Dinner: Spinach and Mushroom Omelet

Snack: Baked Sweet Potato Chips

Dessert: Chocolate Mousse

Day 19:

Breakfast: Veggie Breakfast Burrito

Lunch: Fusilli Salad with Avocado

Dinner: Turkey and Vegetable Skillet

Snack: Zucchini and Corn Fritters

Dessert: Pears with Honey and Cinnamon

Day 20:

Breakfast: Cinnamon Apple Cakes

Lunch: Tuna Salad with Feta Cheese and Spinach

Dinner: Grilled Balsamic Pork Chops with Greek Style Stuffed Mushrooms

Snack: Raspberry Chia Jam

Dessert: Carrot Cake Muffins


Day 21:

Breakfast: Oatmeal with Fresh Berries

Lunch: Shrimp Noodles with Veggies

Dinner: Spinach and Mushroom Omelet

Snack: Baked Sweet Potato Chips

Dessert: Chocolate Mousse

# Week 4

Breakfast: Apple Cinnamon Overnight Oat

Lunch: Delicious Cod Sandwich

Dinner: Shrimp and Asparagus Stir Fry with Herb Cauliflower Rice

Snack: Chocolate Banana Morsels

Dessert: Honeydew Lime Sorbet

Breakfast: Baked Eggs with Veggies

Lunch: Easy Quinoa Salad

Dinner: Beef Kabobs with Pepper

Snack: Apple and Almond Butter Wraps

Dessert: Lemon Yoghurt Cake

Day 24:

Breakfast: Berry Smoothie

Lunch: Grilled Lemon Herb Tofu with Roasted Vegetables

Dinner: Lemon Garlic Shrimp Skewers with Quinoa Salad

Snack: Cucumber Roll-Ups

Dessert: Cinnamon Rice Cakes

Day 25:

Breakfast: Veggie Breakfast Burrito

Lunch: Fusilli Salad with Avocado

Dinner: Turkey and Vegetable Skillet

Snack: Zucchini and Corn Fritters

Dessert: Pears with Honey and Cinnamon

Day 26:

Breakfast: Greek Yogurt with Honey and Nuts

Lunch: Chickpea Salad with Vegetables

Dinner: Baked Cod with Lemon Caper Sauce and Herb Cauliflower Rice

Snack: Blueberry Oat Muffins

Dessert: Pineapple Coconut Smoothie


Day 27:

Breakfast: Cinnamon Apple Cakes

Lunch: Tuna Salad with Feta Cheese and Spinach

Dinner: Grilled Balsamic Pork Chops with Greek Style Stuffed Mushrooms

Snack: Raspberry Chia Jam

Dessert: Carrot Cake Muffins

Day 28:

Breakfast: Ham and Cheese Omelet

Lunch: Seafood Pasta with Tomatoes

Dinner: Baked Cod with Roasted Vegetables

Snack: Carrot and Ginger Soup

Dessert: Strawberry Frozen Yoghurt


Day 29:

Breakfast: Toast with Avocado and Eggs

Lunch: Grilled Vegetable Skewers

Dinner: Pasta with Beef

Snack: Blueberry and Oat Cake

Dessert: Strawberry Frozen Yoghurt


Day 30:

Breakfast: Egg and Vegetable Muffins

Lunch: Fresh Pasta Salad with Vegetables

Dinner: Lemon Yoghurt Cake

Snack: Turkey Lettuce Wraps

Dessert: Peach Crumble

# CONCLUSION

In conclusion, this Chronic Kidney Disease (CKD) Cookbook for Seniors is a guide to improved health and wellbeing, not just a list of recipes. Designed especially for people with chronic kidney disease (CKD), these thoughtfully prepared meals satisfy all the nutritional requirements without sacrificing flavor.

It is impossible to overestimate the importance of following this CKD diet. Seniors who adopt these healthy recipes are not only making smart gastronomic decisions, but they are also actively participating in their own health management. Every ingredient and cooking technique is a purposeful selection to enhance overall vitality and kidney function.

Your health is a journey, dear reader, and this cookbook is your reliable companion. Take inspiration from it to discover the many delectable options available to you while adhering to the restrictions of a CKD diet. You are making an investment in your own health with each carefully planned meal. Always keep in mind that tiny adjustments made today can result in big gains tomorrow.

Therefore, let this CKD Cookbook serve as a source of inspiration rather than just a reference in the kitchen. Using these recipes to commit to your health is a potent form of self-care. You are feeding not only your body but also your soul with every bite. Making the decision to change your health is the first step, and this cookbook will support you every step of the way. Cheers to your health, energy, and many delicious, kidney-friendly meals to come!

## My Little Request

Dear Reader,

Thanks for your purchase, hope you enjoyed reading.

Could you please take a few seconds to leave a positive feedback on this book?

It'll help reach more people and we can collectively help reverse this deadly disease.

Thank you.

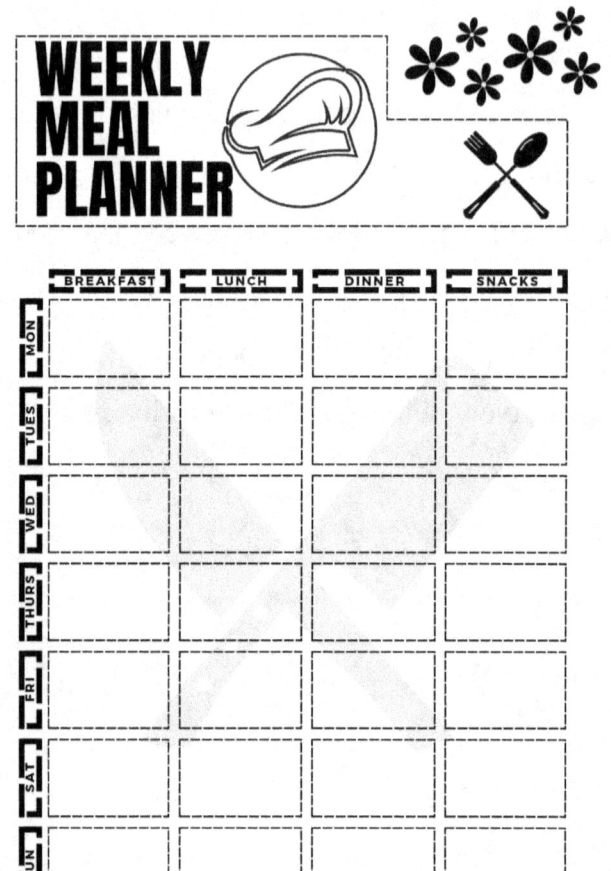

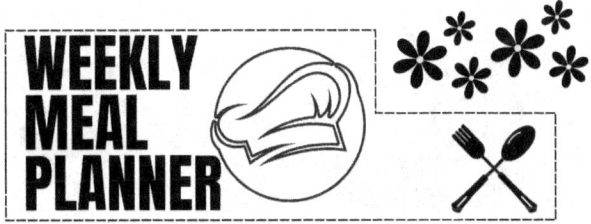

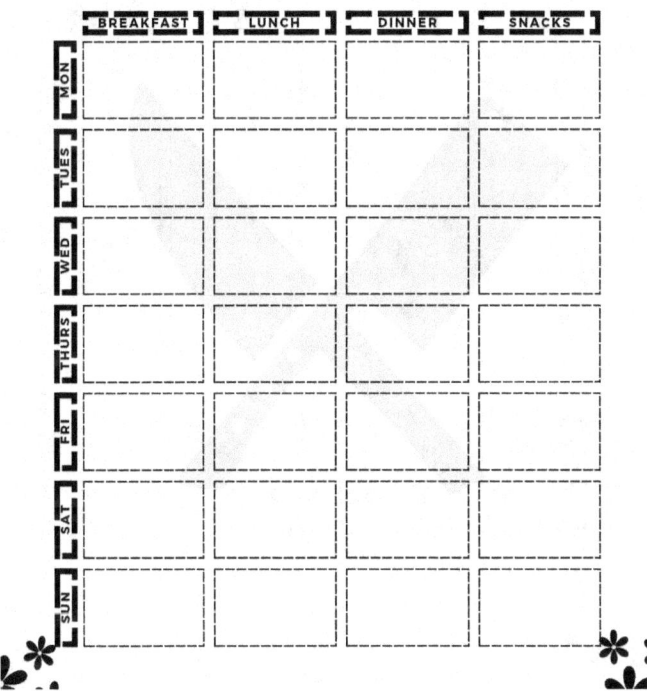

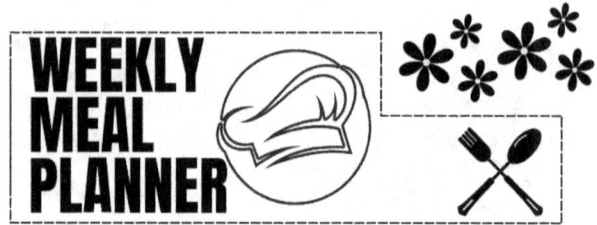

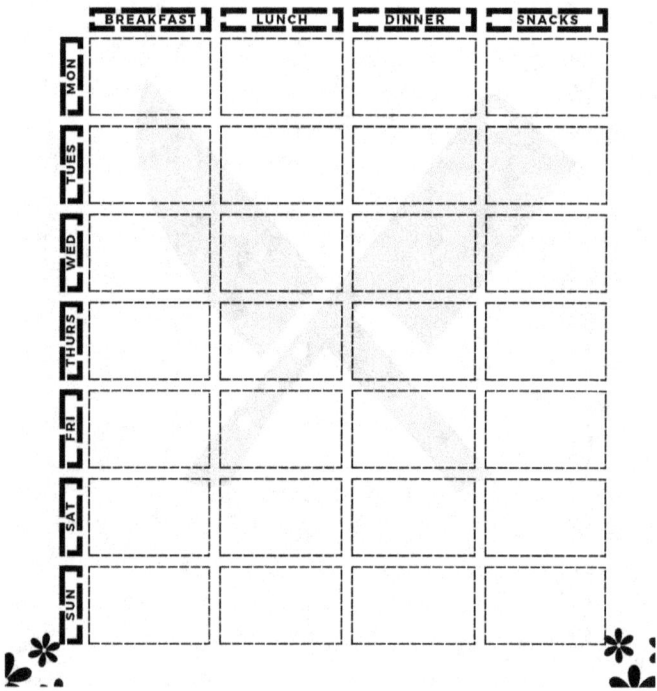

| | BREAKFAST | LUNCH | DINNER | SNACKS |
|---|---|---|---|---|
| MON | | | | |
| TUES | | | | |
| WED | | | | |
| THURS | | | | |
| FRI | | | | |
| SAT | | | | |
| SUN | | | | |

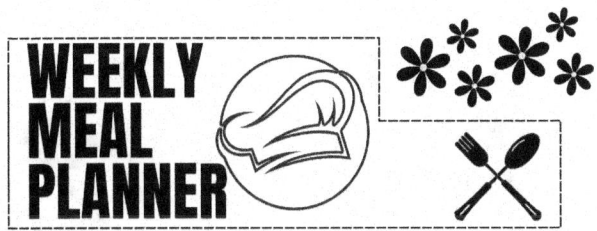

# WEEKLY MEAL PLANNER

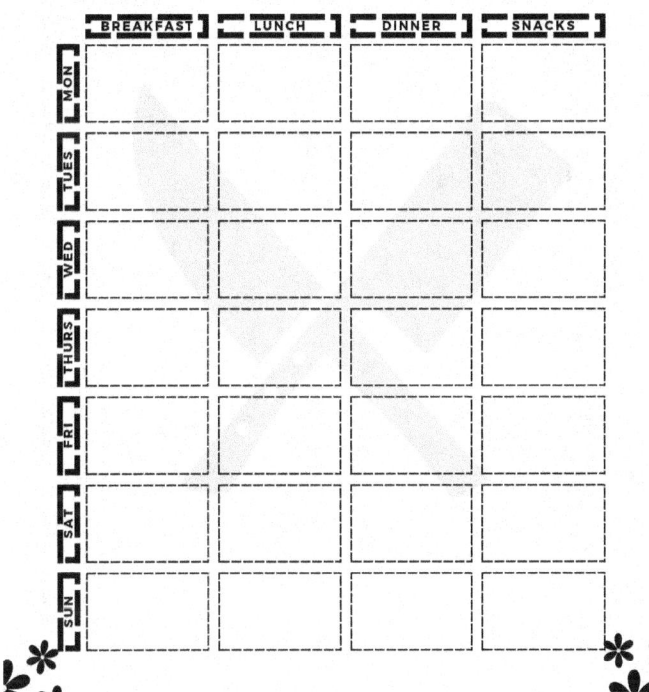

| | BREAKFAST | LUNCH | DINNER | SNACKS |
|---|---|---|---|---|
| MON | | | | |
| TUES | | | | |
| WED | | | | |
| THURS | | | | |
| FRI | | | | |
| SAT | | | | |
| SUN | | | | |

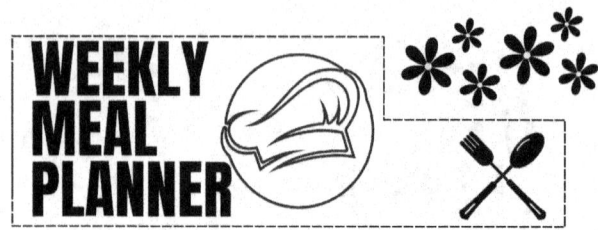

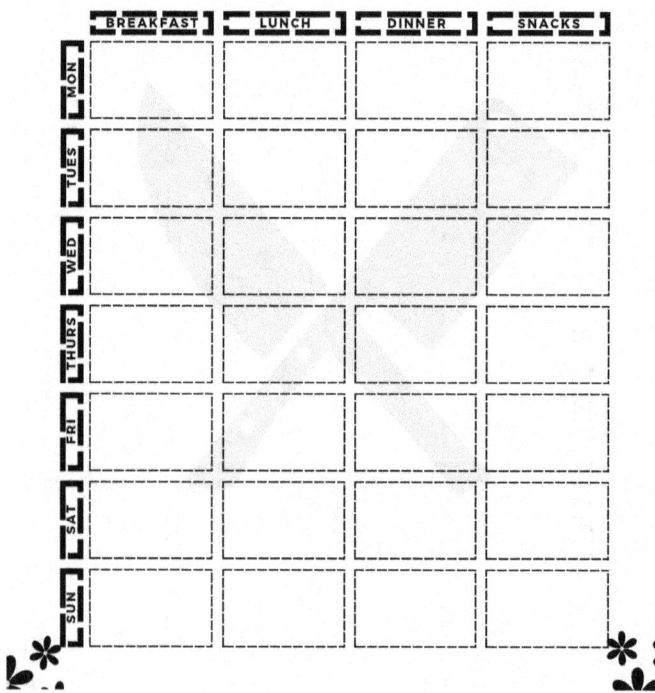

| | BREAKFAST | LUNCH | DINNER | SNACKS |
|---|---|---|---|---|
| MON | | | | |
| TUES | | | | |
| WED | | | | |
| THURS | | | | |
| FRI | | | | |
| SAT | | | | |
| SUN | | | | |

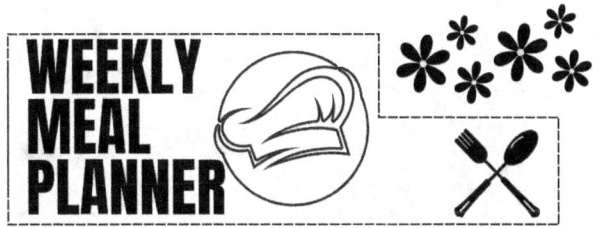

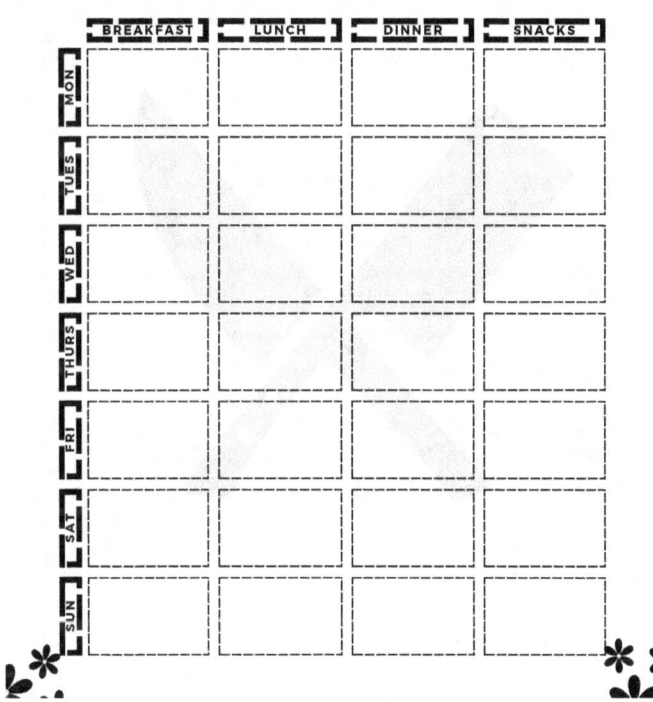

| | BREAKFAST | LUNCH | DINNER | SNACKS |
|---|---|---|---|---|
| MON | | | | |
| TUES | | | | |
| WED | | | | |
| THURS | | | | |
| FRI | | | | |
| SAT | | | | |
| SUN | | | | |

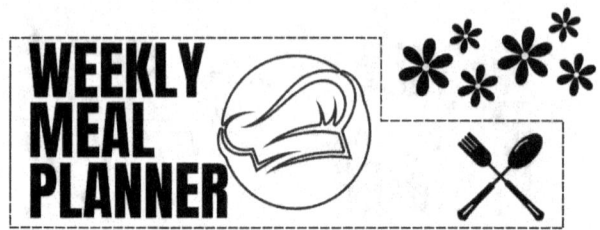

# WEEKLY MEAL PLANNER

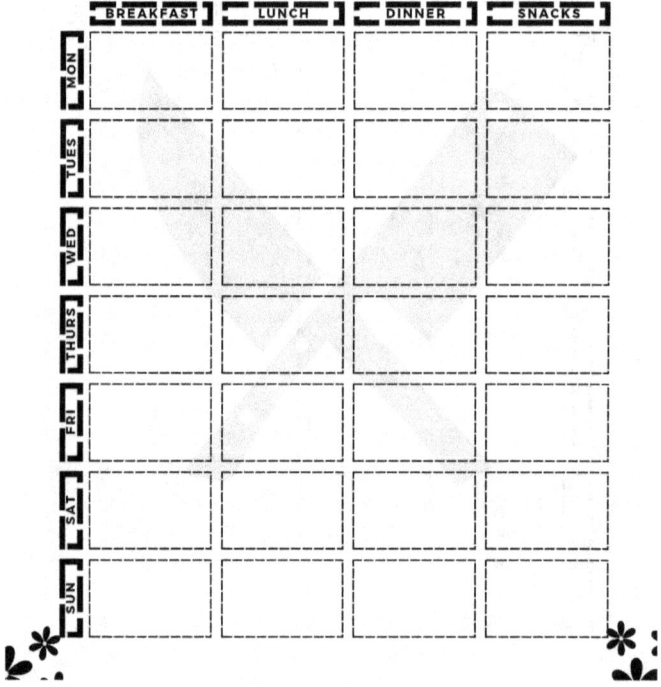

| | BREAKFAST | LUNCH | DINNER | SNACKS |
|---|---|---|---|---|
| MON | | | | |
| TUES | | | | |
| WED | | | | |
| THURS | | | | |
| FRI | | | | |
| SAT | | | | |
| SUN | | | | |

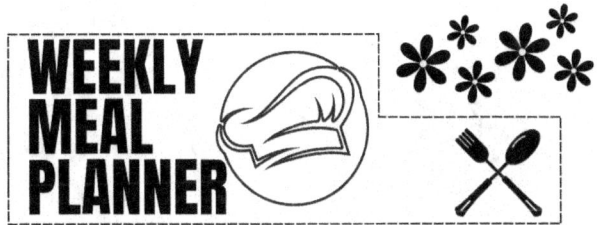

|  | BREAKFAST | LUNCH | DINNER | SNACKS |
|---|---|---|---|---|
| MON | | | | |
| TUES | | | | |
| WED | | | | |
| THURS | | | | |
| FRI | | | | |
| SAT | | | | |
| SUN | | | | |

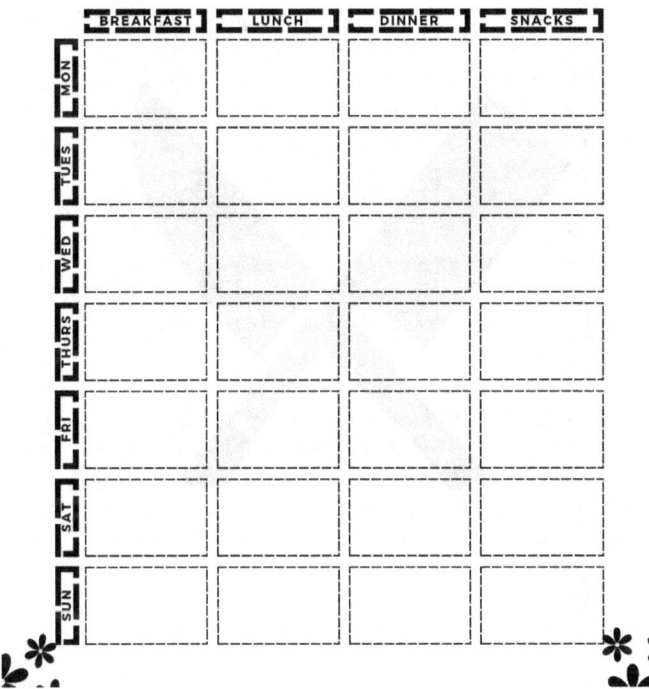

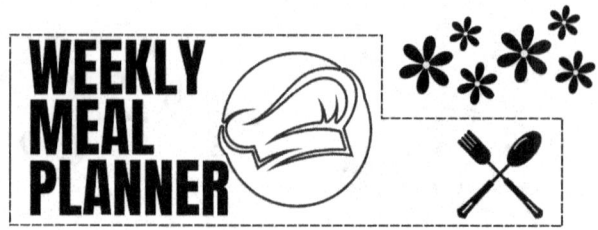

# WEEKLY MEAL PLANNER

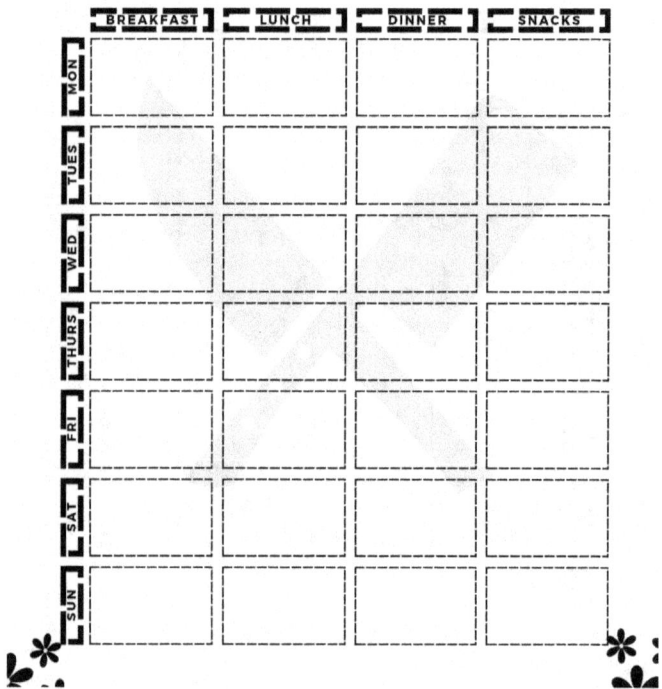

| | BREAKFAST | LUNCH | DINNER | SNACKS |
|---|---|---|---|---|
| MON | | | | |
| TUES | | | | |
| WED | | | | |
| THURS | | | | |
| FRI | | | | |
| SAT | | | | |
| SUN | | | | |

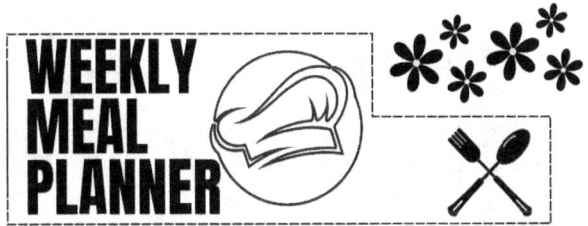

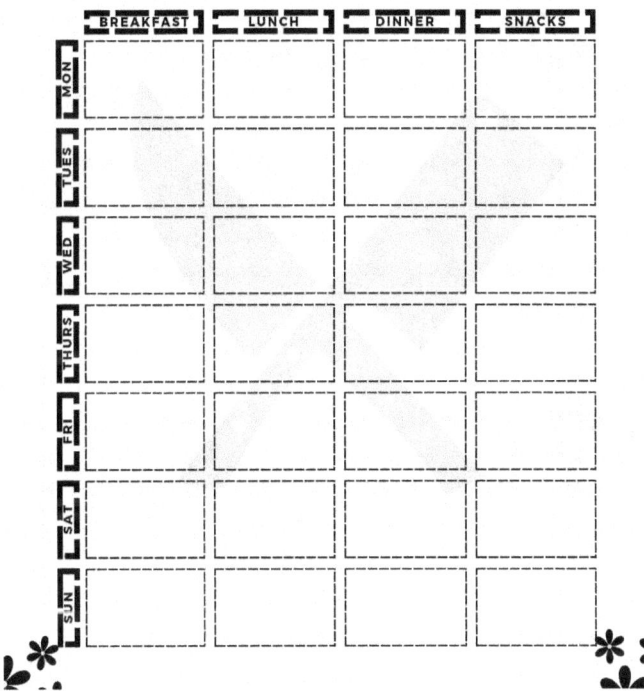

| | BREAKFAST | LUNCH | DINNER | SNACKS |
|---|---|---|---|---|
| MON | | | | |
| TUES | | | | |
| WED | | | | |
| THURS | | | | |
| FRI | | | | |
| SAT | | | | |
| SUN | | | | |

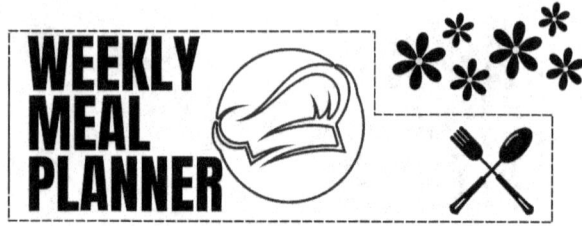

# WEEKLY MEAL PLANNER

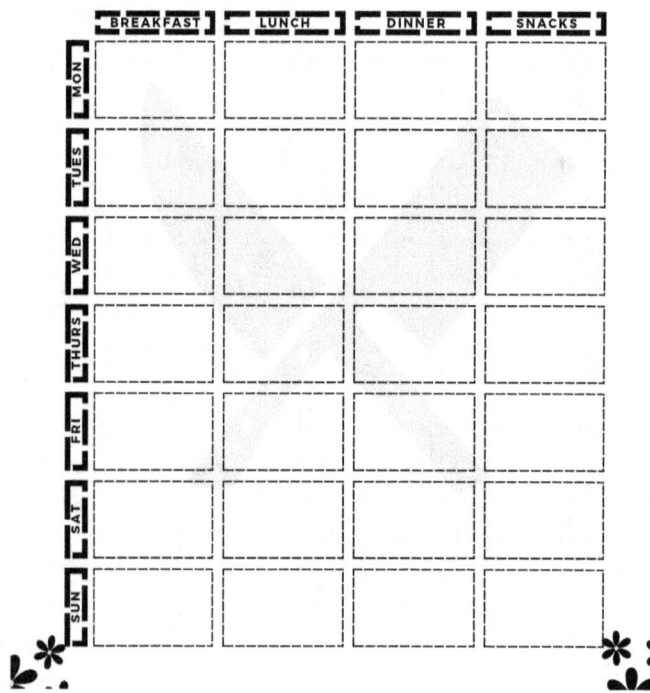

| | BREAKFAST | LUNCH | DINNER | SNACKS |
|---|---|---|---|---|
| MON | | | | |
| TUES | | | | |
| WED | | | | |
| THURS | | | | |
| FRI | | | | |
| SAT | | | | |
| SUN | | | | |

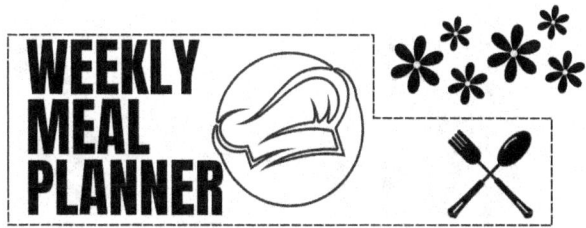

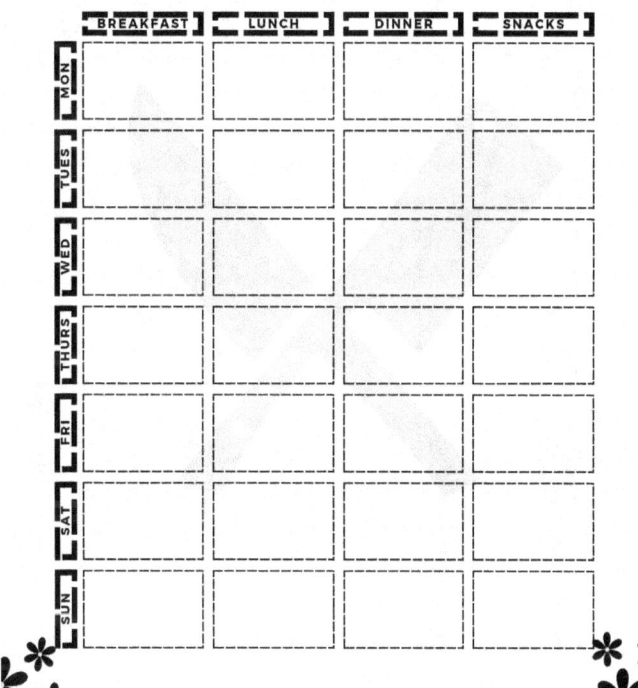

BREAKFAST | LUNCH | DINNER | SNACKS

MON
TUES
WED
THURS
FRI
SAT
SUN

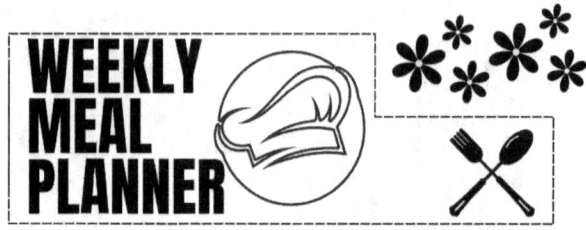

# WEEKLY MEAL PLANNER

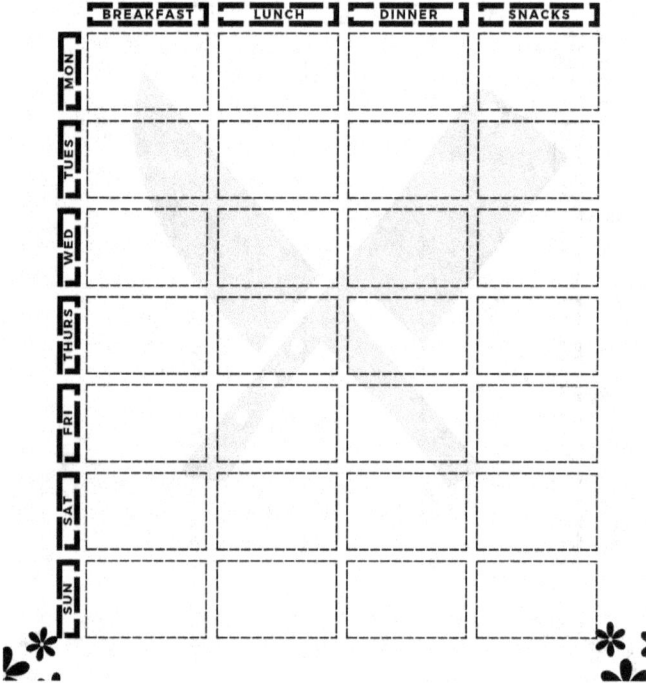

| | BREAKFAST | LUNCH | DINNER | SNACKS |
|---|---|---|---|---|
| MON | | | | |
| TUES | | | | |
| WED | | | | |
| THURS | | | | |
| FRI | | | | |
| SAT | | | | |
| SUN | | | | |

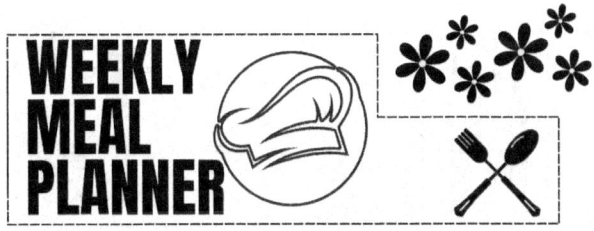

# WEEKLY MEAL PLANNER

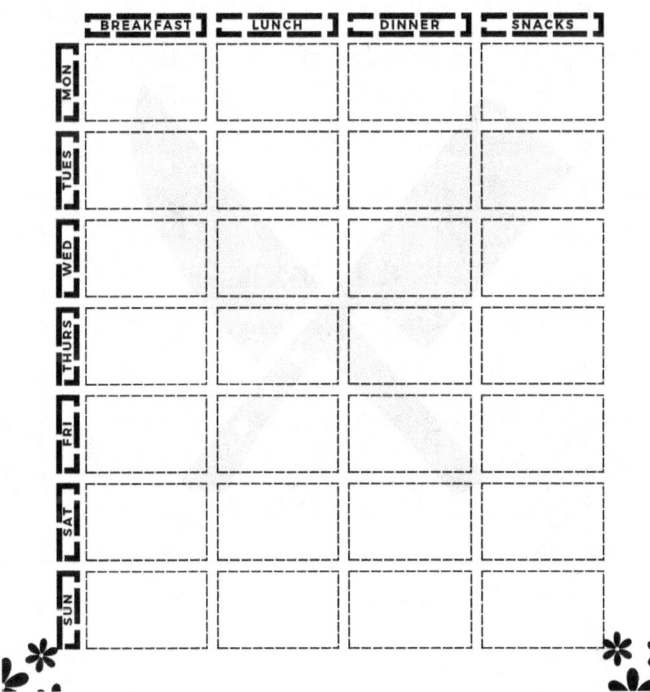

| | BREAKFAST | LUNCH | DINNER | SNACKS |
|---|---|---|---|---|
| MON | | | | |
| TUES | | | | |
| WED | | | | |
| THURS | | | | |
| FRI | | | | |
| SAT | | | | |
| SUN | | | | |

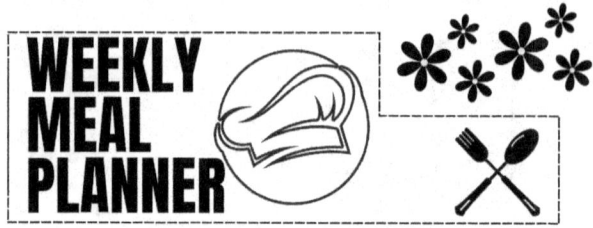

# WEEKLY MEAL PLANNER

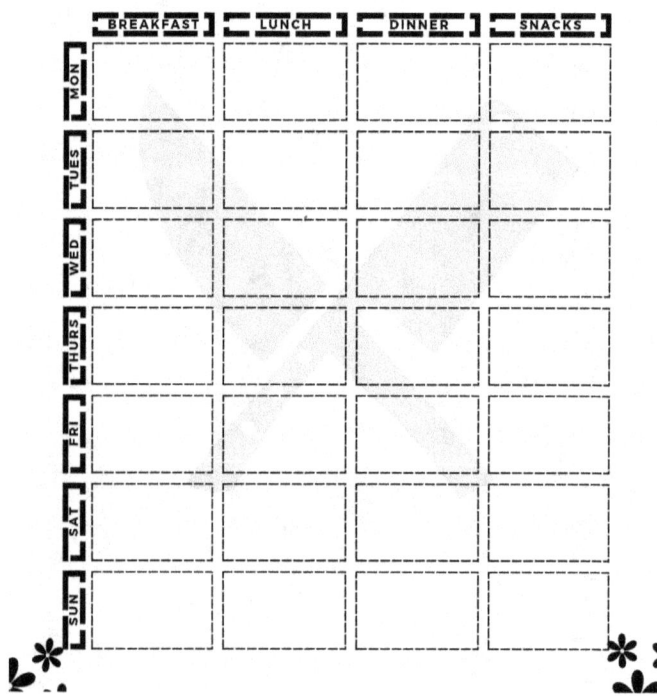

| | BREAKFAST | LUNCH | DINNER | SNACKS |
|---|---|---|---|---|
| MON | | | | |
| TUES | | | | |
| WED | | | | |
| THURS | | | | |
| FRI | | | | |
| SAT | | | | |
| SUN | | | | |

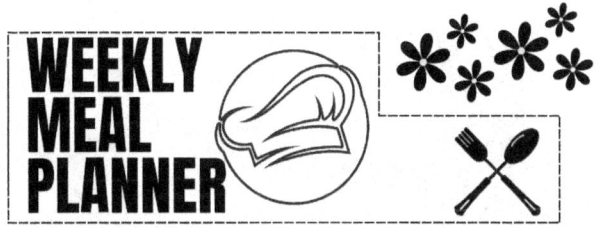

| | BREAKFAST | LUNCH | DINNER | SNACKS |
|---|---|---|---|---|
| MON | | | | |
| TUES | | | | |
| WED | | | | |
| THURS | | | | |
| FRI | | | | |
| SAT | | | | |
| SUN | | | | |

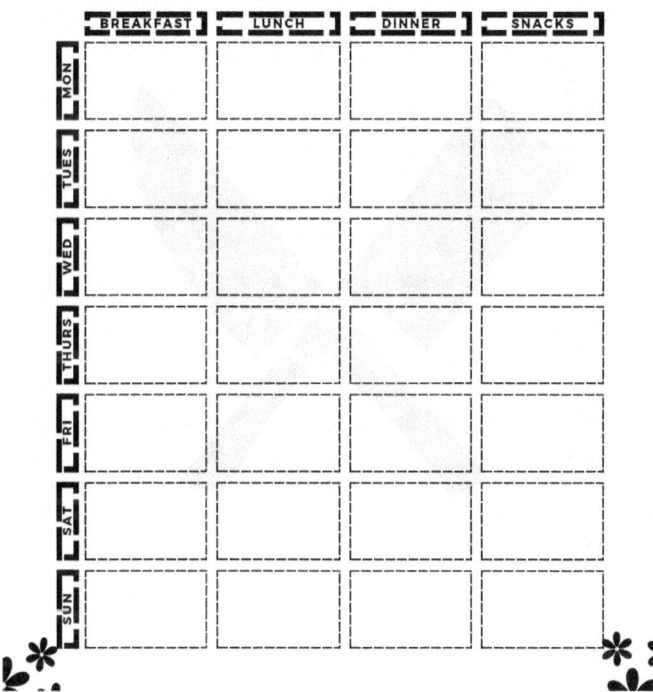

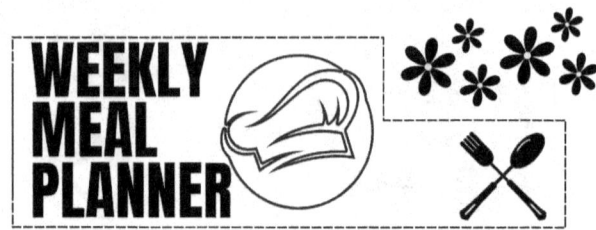

# WEEKLY MEAL PLANNER

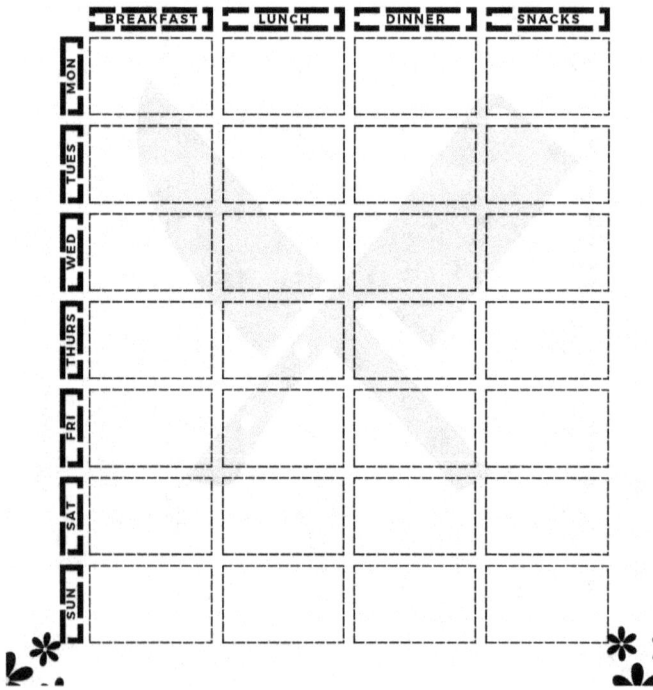

| | BREAKFAST | LUNCH | DINNER | SNACKS |
|---|---|---|---|---|
| MON | | | | |
| TUES | | | | |
| WED | | | | |
| THURS | | | | |
| FRI | | | | |
| SAT | | | | |
| SUN | | | | |

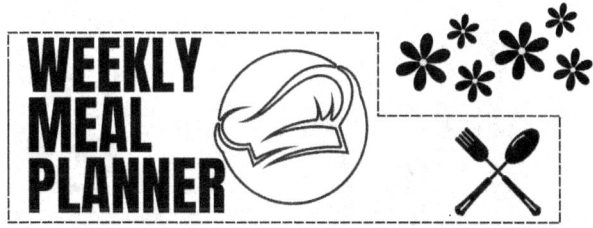

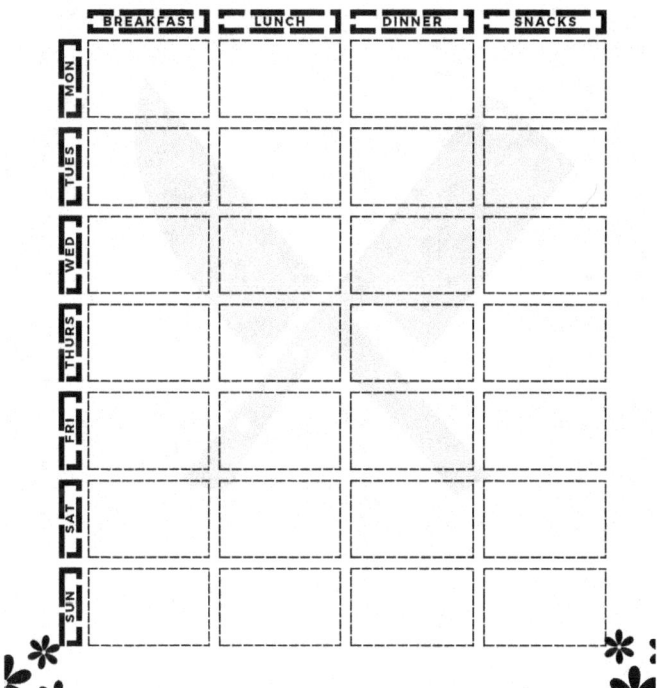

| | BREAKFAST | LUNCH | DINNER | SNACKS |
|---|---|---|---|---|
| MON | | | | |
| TUES | | | | |
| WED | | | | |
| THURS | | | | |
| FRI | | | | |
| SAT | | | | |
| SUN | | | | |

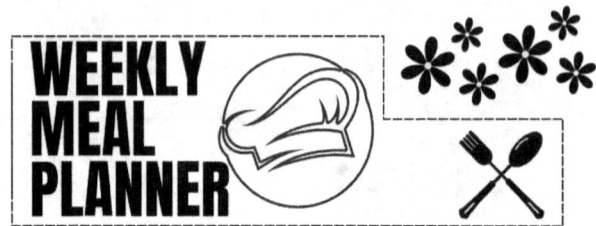

# WEEKLY MEAL PLANNER

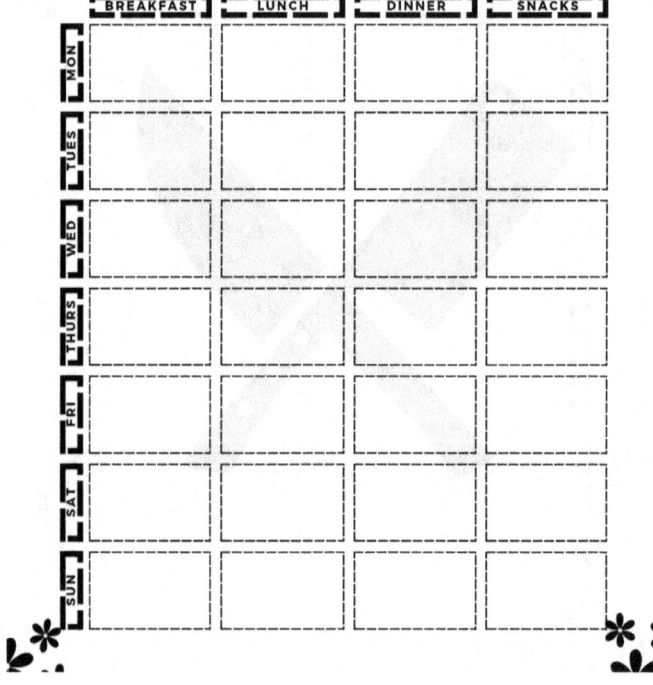

|  | BREAKFAST | LUNCH | DINNER | SNACKS |
|---|---|---|---|---|
| MON | | | | |
| TUES | | | | |
| WED | | | | |
| THURS | | | | |
| FRI | | | | |
| SAT | | | | |
| SUN | | | | |

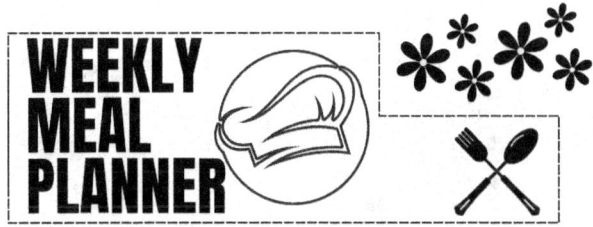

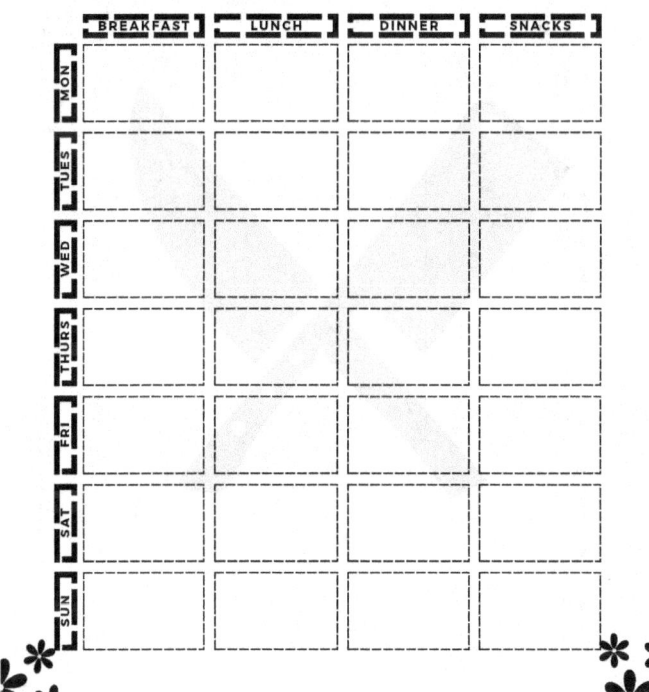

| | BREAKFAST | LUNCH | DINNER | SNACKS |
|---|---|---|---|---|
| MON | | | | |
| TUES | | | | |
| WED | | | | |
| THURS | | | | |
| FRI | | | | |
| SAT | | | | |
| SUN | | | | |

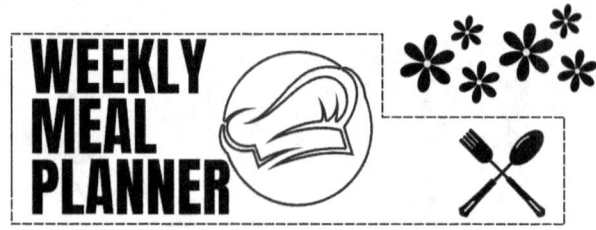

# WEEKLY MEAL PLANNER

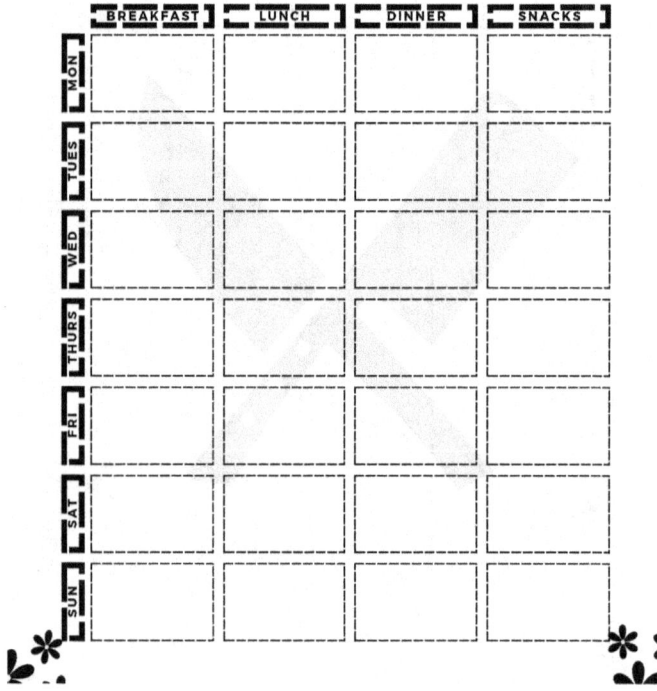

| | BREAKFAST | LUNCH | DINNER | SNACKS |
|---|---|---|---|---|
| MON | | | | |
| TUES | | | | |
| WED | | | | |
| THURS | | | | |
| FRI | | | | |
| SAT | | | | |
| SUN | | | | |

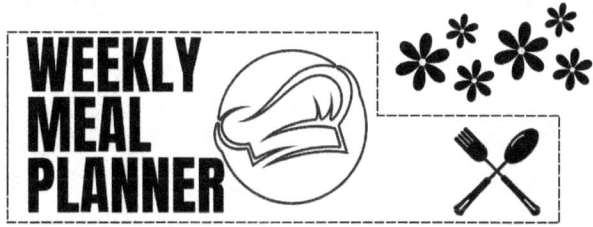

# WEEKLY MEAL PLANNER

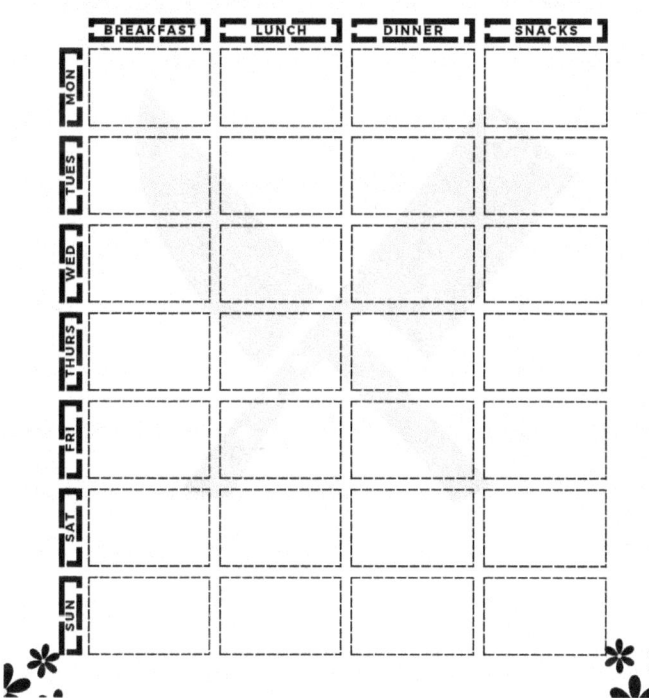

| | BREAKFAST | LUNCH | DINNER | SNACKS |
|---|---|---|---|---|
| MON | | | | |
| TUES | | | | |
| WED | | | | |
| THURS | | | | |
| FRI | | | | |
| SAT | | | | |
| SUN | | | | |

www.ingramcontent.com/pod-product-compliance
Lightning Source LLC
Chambersburg PA
CBHW071044290526
45795CB00004B/1305